Healthcare Public Health

Healthcare Public Health

Improving Health Services Through
Population Science

Edited by

Martin Gulliford

Professor of Public Health, King's College London, UK

Edmund Jessop

Honorary Professor of Public Health, King's College London, UK

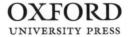

OXFORD
UNIVERSITY PRESS

Great Clarendon Street, Oxford, OX2 6DP,
United Kingdom

Oxford University Press is a department of the University of Oxford.
It furthers the University's objective of excellence in research, scholarship,
and education by publishing worldwide. Oxford is a registered trade mark of
Oxford University Press in the UK and in certain other countries

Published in the United States of America by Oxford University Press
198 Madison Avenue, New York, NY 10016, United States of America

British Library Cataloguing in Publication Data

Data available

Library of Congress Control Number: 2020938109

ISBN 978–0–19–883720–6

Printed and bound by
CPI Group (UK) Ltd, Croydon, CR0 4YY

Contents

Contributors

Hugh Alderwick
Assistant Director of Policy, The Health Foundation, London, UK

Jo Bibby
Director of Health, The Health Foundation, London, UK

Bo Burström
Professor and Senior Consultant in Social Medicine, Department of Public Health Sciences, Karolinska Institutet, Sweden

Jennifer Dixon
Chief Executive, The Health Foundation, London, UK

Rhiannon Tudor Edwards
Professor in Health Economics, Centre for Health Economics and Medicines Research (CHEME), Bangor University, UK

Nina Fudge
Research Associate, Institute of Population Health Sciences, Barts and the London School of Medicine and Dentistry, Queen Mary University of London, UK

Martin Gulliford
Professor of Public Health, School of Population Health and Environmental Sciences, King's College London, UK

Matthew Harris
Clinical Senior Lecturer in Public Health, Faculty of Medicine, School of Public Health, Imperial College London, UK

Nehmat Houssami
Professor of Public Health, Faculty of Medicine and Health, University of Sydney, Australia

Edmund Jessop
Honorary Professor of Public Health, King's College London, UK; Public Health Adviser, NHS and Public Health England, UK

James Mapstone
Acting Regional Director, Public Health England, UK

Christopher McKevitt
Professor of Social Science & Health, School of Population Health and Environmental Sciences, King's College London, UK

Aoife Molloy
Research Postgraduate, Faculty of Medicine, Department of Surgery & Cancer, Imperial College London, UK

Andrew O'Shaughnessy
Consultant in Public Health, Bradford City Council, UK

Clémence Pinel
Postdoctoral Researcher, Department of Public Health, University of Copenhagen, Denmark

Stephanie Russ
NIHR Knowledge Mobilisation Research Fellow in Patient Safety, Centre for Implementation Science, King's College London, UK

Julio Cesar Schweickardt
Head of the Laboratory for the History, Public Policy and Health in the Amazon region, Oswaldo Cruz Foundation, Brazil

Nick Sevdalis
Professor of Implementation Science & Patient Safety, Director of the Centre for Implementation Science, King's College London, UK

Jenifer Smith
Programme Director, Public Health
England, UK

Allison Streetly
Deputy National Lead, Healthcare Public
Health, Public Health England, UK; Senior
Lecturer, Department of Population Health
Sciences, King's College London, UK

Rodrigo Tobias
Researcher, Laboratory for the History,
Public Policy and Health in the Amazon re-
gion, Leonidas and Maria Deane Institute,
Oswalda Cruz Foundation, Brazil

A.M. Viens
Associate Professor in Global Health Policy,
Faculty of Health, York University, Canada

Eira Winrow
Research Officer in Health Economics,
Centre for Health Economics and Medicines
Research (CHEME), Bangor University, UK

John Wright
Director of Research, Bradford Institute for
Health Research, UK

Lucy Yardley
Professor of Health Psychology, University of
Bristol and University of Southampton, UK

1

Healthcare public health

An introduction

Martin Gulliford and Edmund Jessop

1.1 Definitions

Public health represents 'the art and science of preventing disease, prolonging life and promoting health through the organized efforts of society' (Acheson, 1988). The public health community has traditionally considered the main role of health services to be the relief of sickness and suffering, rather than the production of health and promotion of longevity (McKeown, 1979), but this view is no longer tenable. Medical care accounted for about half of the seven-year increase in life expectancy in the USA between 1960 and 2000 (Cutler et al., 2006). Since then there have been even more substantial reductions in mortality from cardiovascular diseases (Mensah et al., 2017) and cancer (Allemani et al., 2018). Basic, clinical, and public health sciences have transformed human immunodeficiency virus (HIV) infection from a condition that could not be diagnosed or treated, to one with greatly increased survival, through antiretroviral treatment (Global Burden of Disease Study, 2016). In middle- and low-income countries, vaccines represent some of the most cost-effective interventions and have a major impact on child survival, offering the prospect of eliminating important vaccine-preventable diseases. We can now be confident that health services have the potential to have a major impact on population health. The role of healthcare public health and population healthcare is to ensure that this potential is fulfilled.

Drawing on Acheson's definition of public health quoted earlier, we can define healthcare public health as 'the art and science of preventing disease, prolonging life, and promoting health through the organization and delivery of population-wide health services'. Healthcare public health is one of three main domains of public health, alongside health protection and health improvement. Health protection is concerned with the control of communicable diseases and other environmental hazards, while health improvement addresses the impact of broader determinants of health. Healthcare public health draws on knowledge from the basic sciences. It also draws on epidemiology and other social sciences. However, it also requires skills in judging how to value conflicting objectives, involving patients, and engaging with communities and the wider public, advocating the population health perspective to politicians and policy makers. Some of the key activities in healthcare public health are outlined in Box 1.1.

Martin Gulliford and Edmund Jessop, *Healthcare public health* In: *Healthcare Public Health*. Edited by: Martin Gulliford and Edmund Jessop, Oxford University Press (2020). © Oxford University Press. DOI: 10.1093/oso/9780198837206.003.0001.

Box 1.1 Main activities in healthcare public health

- Designing effective and efficient health and social care interventions, settings, and pathways of care
- Facilitating access and meeting the needs of all individuals and groups
- Maximizing the population benefits of healthcare
- Preventing disease
- Improving health-related outcomes
- Reducing health inequalities
- Prioritizing available resources

Source: data from UK Faculty of Public Health (2017) *Short Headline Definition of Healthcare Public Health*. London: Faculty of Public Health. Available at https://www.fph.org.uk/media/1879/hcph-definition-final.pdf

---

1.2 Classifying healthcare interventions

Initially, we can consider the impact of healthcare interventions on health outcomes and healthcare resource use at the aggregate level. The cost-effectiveness plane (Figure 1.1) enables us to classify healthcare interventions into four groups. The upper left quadrant (A in Figure 1.1) includes interventions that result in increased costs but reduced health status. It seems clear that interventions of this type should not be employed. But every time a practitioner orders an unnecessary test or prescribes a potentially unneeded treatment, resource use may be

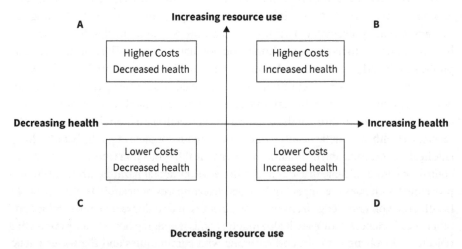

Figure 1.1 Cost-effectiveness plane.

increased and harms may result. UK general practitioners prescribe antibiotics at more than 50% of consultations for self-limiting respiratory infections (Gulliford et al., 2014), even though these are generally caused by viruses. Patients do not benefit from this treatment and often experience side effects; there are also wider community impacts from antimicrobial resistance (O'Neill et al., 2016). There is a significant public health role in identifying and eradicating these harmful clinical practices.

The lower right quadrant (D in Figure 1.1) identifies interventions that, when compared to current practice, are associated with improved health status and reduced resource use. These interventions should be employed to the maximum extent possible. A recent systematic review found that preventive interventions including falls prevention programmes, needle exchange schemes, and smoking cessation programmes fall into this category (Masters et al., 2017). Public health specialists should advocate for these interventions, but only after carefully scrutinizing the evidence on which claims are based, including both the scope and time horizons for estimation of costs. Many preventive medical interventions yield benefits over long time horizons, while costs may be incurred immediately. Despite their cost effectiveness, these interventions may sometimes be challenging to justify to decision makers when set against the immediate needs of acutely ill patients.

Much public health work is concerned with interventions that fall into the upper right quadrant (B in Figure 1.1), where costs are increased and health outcomes are improved. Investment in these interventions may be justified by the health benefits obtained. For many decisions, it makes sense to rank these interventions in terms of the cost per unit health outcome obtained, employing a metric that can be compared across interventions with such as the cost per quality adjusted life year (QALY), advocating for increased use of procedures with more favourable incremental cost-effectiveness ratios.

The lower left quadrant (C in Figure 1.1) is concerned with interventions that might save resources but at the price of worse health outcomes. Initially, it might appear that interventions of this type could not be ethically justified because of the harm that could result to patients. Yet, suppose the 'intervention' represented disinvestment from a high-cost procedure; suppose, too, that the resources saved could be allocated to lower-cost procedures that could be associated with greater health gains. Then, an ethical argument could be made for justifying this approach. The opportunity cost of a high-cost procedure may not be justifiable if less costly interventions might yield greater health gains. A threshold of £30,000 per QALY is often used to judge whether an intervention is cost effective in the UK. If disinvestment or some other intervention might save more than £30,000 per QALY, then this might be justified. This discussion raises important ethical questions about how resource allocation questions should be answered: Who should be responsible for taking such decisions? What is a fair procedure for decision making?

1.3 Health and healthcare distribution and access

As well as considering aggregate costs and benefits, we should consider the share of health and healthcare received by different groups in the population. The Lorenz curve provides one way of evaluating inequality. Figure 1.2 illustrates inequality according to one socioeconomic measure, household income. The horizontal axis represents the cumulative proportion of the population ranked by household income, while the vertical axis represents the cumulative proportion of health or healthcare received. The solid line represents a condition of equality, where each group in the population receives the same share of health or healthcare regardless of their income. In reality, lower-income groups have a smaller share of health, while higher-income groups have a larger share of population health. This pro-rich inequality is shown in the dotted line in Figure 1.2. The dashed line in Figure 1.2 represents the cumulative share of primary healthcare that each group receives. In this simulated example, there is a pro-poor distribution of primary care utilization consistent with the increased utilization of primary care that is commonly observed among lower socioeconomic groups in high-income countries (van Doorslaer et al., 2006). The situation differs with respect to specialist care, with higher-income groups receiving a larger share, consistent with pro-rich inequity (van Doorslaer et al., 2006). This is a manifestation of the inverse care law, which Tudor Hart (2000) described. This is shown in the dot–dashed line in Figure 1.2.

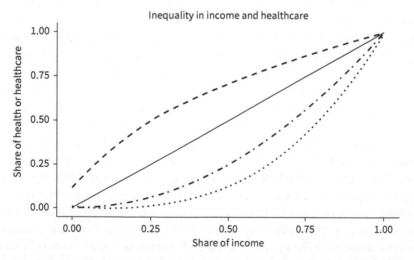

Figure 1.2 Lorenz curve showing the cumulative distribution of health (dotted line), cumulative utilization of primary healthcare (dashed line), cumulative utilization of specialist care (dot–dash line), plotted against cumulative share of income.

Evaluating inequalities in health and healthcare access, and identifying actions to reduce inequalities, are key elements in healthcare public health. Fairness would appear to require that the healthcare utilization of lower-income groups should be in proportion to their greater health needs, but how can health needs be defined and measured? What distribution of healthcare is fair?

These considerations shift our attention from the costs and outcomes of clinical interventions towards the design of care pathways and systems of care that can act as delivery platforms to ensure that timely and coordinated services can be delivered to all who need them. Vaccines are highly cost-effective interventions, but ensuring adequate coverage of the population at risk requires a delivery system that includes adequately staffed primary care clinics in accessible locations, with convenient opening hours, and a secure supply of vaccines. Vaccines may be regarded as too dangerous to use by some groups, and even as an enemy action in some conflict zones, reminding us that public health programmes are located in a social and political environment which may need our attention.

Even when there is a well-organized system of primary care, the needs of marginalized groups may not always be visible, and delivery of services to these groups requires special consideration. Homeless people, new migrants, or people with serious mental health disorders may not be able to articulate their needs, nor gain access to medical services that they might benefit from, because of a combination of financial, legal, administrative, and social barriers to accessing care (Abarca Tomas et al., 2013). This may be indicative of a mismatch between the design of services and the needs and perceptions of the people they are intended to serve. This kind of mismatch can also arise from changing population characteristics over time. In high-income countries, very old people (aged more than 80 years) represent the fastest growing sector of the population, and this group includes high users of health services. Health services need to adapt to the health needs of a frail population with multiple impairments and morbidities, with supporting care at home and in community settings in addition to traditionally structured hospital care.

1.4 Structure of this volume

The chapters in this volume analyse these issues for population healthcare in greater depth. Rodrigo Tobias and colleagues describe the challenges of delivering population healthcare in one remote and resource-poor region, the Brazilian Amazon. Bo Burström discusses some of the challenges of promoting equity in health services in a high-income country, Sweden. The following chapter by Christopher McKevitt and colleagues discusses patient and public involvement in health services. Adrian Viens then analyses ethical questions in population healthcare, showing how the contrasting perspectives of individuals and populations need to be reconciled. The next five chapters outline the core methods of healthcare public health: healthcare needs' assessment by Andrew O'Shaughnessy and John Wright; facilitating access to healthcare by Martin Gulliford; managing new knowledge to improve population health by Aoife Molloy; designing new services by Hugh Alderwick and colleagues; and developing a business case by Eira Winrow and Rhiannon Tudor Edwards. The following chapter by Edmund Jessop then outlines approaches to evaluation of health services. Stephanie Russ and Nick Sevdalis then show how new scientific approaches can be used to analyse and enhance patient safety and improve service quality. In the remaining chapters, Jenifer Smith and James Mapstone provide an overview of the role of health services in disease prevention intervention; Allison Streetly and Nehmat Houssami describe population-screening strategies; and we, together with Lucy Yardley, consider the potential of digital technologies for healthcare public health. The Coronavirus pandemic has drawn attention to the importance of health services in emergencies. Edmund Jessop outlines the principles of responding to disasters and emergencies.

We aim to provide an introduction to the methods and subject matter of healthcare public health to enable future students, researchers and practitioners to contribute to the goal of designing and delivering health services that improve population health, reduce inequalities, and meet the needs of individuals and communities.

References

Abarca Tomas, B., Pell, C., Bueno Cavanillas, A., Guillen Solvas, J., Pool, R., & Roura, M. (2013). Tuberculosis in migrant populations. A systematic review of the qualitative literature. *PLoS One*, 8(12), e82440.

Acheson, E.D. (1988). *Committee of Inquiry into the Future Development of the Public Health Function. Public Health in England.* London: HMSO.

Allemani, C., et al. (2018). Global surveillance of trends in cancer survival 2000–14 (CONCORD-3): analysis of individual records for 37,513,025 patients diagnosed with one of 18 cancers from 322 population-based registries in 71 countries. *Lancet,* 391(10125), 1023–1075.

Cutler, D.M., Rosen, A.B., & Vijan, S. (2006). The value of medical spending in the United States, 1960–2000. *New Engl J Med,* 355(9), 920–927.

Global Burden of Disease Study. (2016). Estimates of global, regional, and national incidence, prevalence, and mortality of HIV, 1980–2015: the Global Burden of Disease Study 2015. *Lancet HIV,* 3(8), e361–e387.

Gulliford, M.C., et al. (2014). Continued high rates of antibiotic prescribing to adults with respiratory tract infection: survey of 568 UK general practices. *BMJ Open,* 4(10), e006245.

Masters, R., Anwar, E., Collins, B., Cookson, R., & Capewell, S. (2017). Return on investment of public health interventions: a systematic review. *J Epidemiol Comm Health,* 71(8), 827.

McKeown, T. (1979). *The Role of Medicine.* Oxford: Blackwell.

Mensah, G.A., et al. (2017). Decline in cardiovascular mortality. *Circ Res,* 120(2), 366–380.

O'Neill, J., et al. (2016). *The Review on Antimicrobial Resistance Chaired by Jim O'Neill. Tackling Drug-Resistant Infections Globally: Final Report and Recommendations.* London: Review on Antimicrobial Resistance.

Tudor Hart, J. (2000). Commentary: three decades of the inverse care law. *BMJ,* 320(7226), 18–19.

UK Faculty of Public Health. (2017). *Short Headline Definition of Healthcare Public Health*. London: Faculty of Public Health. Available at: https://www.fph.org.uk/media/1879/hcph-definition-final.pdf [accessed 23 July 2019].

van Doorslaer, E., Masseria, C., & Koolman, X. for the OECD Health Equity Research Group. (2006). Inequalities in access to medical care by income in developed countries. *CMAJ*, 174(2), 177–183. Available at: https://www.ncbi.nlm.nih.gov/pmc/articles/PMC1329455/pdf/20060117s00017p177.pdf

2

Access to healthcare in the remote and resource-poor region of the Brazilian Amazon

Rodrigo Tobias, Julio Cesar Schweickardt, and Matthew Harris

2.1 Introduction

Access to healthcare, including primary care, is a particular challenge in low- and middle-income countries. This may be due to a shortage of medical professionals through problems with retention, recruitment, or training; physical barriers to access such as precarious transportation systems or distance; or financial barriers such as fee-for-service payments which can lead to catastrophic out-of-pocket payments when illness strikes. Many low- and middle-income countries have been reforming their health systems to address this important question of healthcare access. The goal to achieve universal healthcare coverage, where citizens have good access to a wide range of comprehensive services at minimal cost to themselves, is a goal that most countries, even wealthy ones, are still grappling with. Brazil has made substantial progress in this regard, predominantly through wholesale reform of its primary care system, the bedrock of its unified health system. This chapter focuses on the particular context of the Amazon region in Brazil as a case study of how to organize services in one of the world's most remote, and inaccessible, regions.

A country with areas of extreme wealth and extreme poverty, Brazil is one of the world's most unequal societies with a Gini Index of 53.3 in 2017 (World Bank, 2019). Healthcare public health, in particular the integration of public health activities into primary care services (Starfield, 2002), is of increasing interest in Brazil. It was only in the 1990s that Brazil developed its national policy on primary care, placing it centrally within the organization of the health system as a whole. Initially known as the Family Health Programme (PSF in Portuguese) and latterly termed the Family Health Strategy (ESF in Portuguese), it has become fully integrated into all spheres of government at national, regional, and municipal levels, and has expanded to cover 95% of all municipalities. The ESF serves 70% of the population (Macinko and Harris, 2015), and is thus in a prime position to deliver significant improvements in public health outcomes (Aquino et al., 2009, 2014).

Rodrigo Tobias, Julio Cesar Schweickardt, and Matthew Harris, *Access to healthcare in the remote and resource-poor region of the Brazilian Amazon* In: *Healthcare Public Health*. Edited by: Martin Gulliford and Edmund Jessop, Oxford University Press (2020). © Oxford University Press. DOI: 10.1093/oso/9780198837206.003.0002.

There is evidence to suggest that the expansion of the ESF, as the principal operating model for primary care delivery throughout the country, has led to significant reductions in inequalities in mortality rates between different ethnic groups (Hone et al., 2017); reduced mortality due to diarrhoea and respiratory illnesses in children less than five years of age (Rasella et al., 2010) and cardiovascular disease (Rasella et al., 2014); and reductions in hospitalizations for ambulatory care-sensitive conditions (Macinko et al., 2010). Macinko et al. (2010) found that in municipalities with high enrolment of the ESF, hospitalizations due to ambulatory care-sensitive conditions were 17% lower than municipalities with low enrolment. Hone et al. (2017) found that ESF expansion (from 0% to 100%) was associated with a 15.4% (95% CI: 10.1% to 20.4%) reduction in mortality from ambulatory care sensitive conditions (ACSCs) in the black/pardo (mixed) group compared with a 6.8% (95% CI: 2.6% to 10.8%) reduction in the white group. In addition, the ESF has been highly efficient in terms of cost. Brazil spends only around $50 per person per annum (Rocha & Soares, 2010) on primary care delivered through the ESF.

In 2017, the Brazilian government reformed the National Primary Care Policy (PNAB, 2017), the principle guiding policy on all matters related to primary care, in order to guarantee its provision in all regions of the country. The fundamental principles of the policy are to 'ensure a prescribed geographical territory to each primary health care team, guarantee continuous, longitudinal care, and to serve a coordinating and integrating role, provide ambulatory care services, stimulate community participation in order to improve autonomy and health literacy, and to engage in the determinants of health and wellbeing' (Brasil, 2017). Critical to this is the importance of developing close ties with, and a sense of responsibility for the public health outcomes of the whole community (Brasil, 2017).

The ESF is the bedrock of the entire national health system, referred to as the Sistema Unica de Saude (SUS). The SUS was established in 1988, as Brazil was emerging from decades of military rule, and was a social, non-partisan, constitutional project to address the health and social inequalities of the entire Brazilian population (Paim, 2015). Part of the operational directives of the SUS is to ensure that healthcare delivery is adapted to the social, economic, and public health realities of the many distinct and diverse regions. This is achieved through the decentralized management of the health system at municipal levels, and federal and state transfer of resources to municipal governments and prefectures. Brazil has 5,560 municipalities and each are responsible for primary care delivery and management. Eight per cent of these are located in the Amazon region, characterized by extreme difficulty in terms of access to healthcare services.

The delivery of integrated and equitable primary healthcare in the Amazon is very challenging. Facilitating access to services needs to take into account what is known as the 'Amazon factor'—the combination of:

(a) large distances;
(b) the use of rivers as the main mode of transport;
(c) significant climatic changes impeding access to many locations for much of the year;

    (d) natural physical barriers such as impenetrable forests; and

    (e) infectious disease outbreaks requiring specific interventions that incorporate health services as well as many other sectors in the local geo-, socio-, and political economy (Lima et al., 2016).

These factors contribute important barriers to accessibility of services organized according to conventional models.

    In order to achieve the fundamental principles of universal, continuous, and longitudinal healthcare provision in a region of this complexity, primary care and public health services need to be reconsidered to take into account the extremely low population density and challenging access and transportation issues. To this end, particular legal frameworks have been incorporated into the PNAB and also the National Policy on Health Care for Indigenous Populations. This chapter addresses the challenge of integrating primary care and public health services in a region of these extremes, with a particular focus on how Brazil meets the challenge of reducing inequalities in access, through particular delivery models and management strategies. Our point of departure is to consider the different 'Amazons' that constitute the Amazon region and how this has fostered debate and analysis between the different administrative levels and societal actors involved in delivery of healthcare public health services.

    We have structured the chapter into four sections. In the first section, we examine the Amazon as a territory, its social relations and networks, and explore the political environment through which health policies are created and delivered. In the second section, we explore the structures and processes of primary care in the Amazon, in particular how services respond to the idea of the 'fluid territory' as an analytical category in public policy. Next, we describe the delivery of primary healthcare in riverside populations and communities, drawing from the experiences of Riverside Health Teams that are based on boats, specially constructed and reconfigured to provide primary care, health promotion, and health protection services. Finally, we examine the national policies surrounding indigenous population health services as a particular element of primary care delivery in specific population groups in the Amazon.

2.2 The context of the Brazilian Amazon

The Brazilian Amazon is one of the largest reservoirs of biological diversity and is a biome characterized by humid tropical rainforest. There is an enormous diversity of cultures, ethnicities, and indigenous languages, with over 900,000 indigenous inhabitants, 305 ethnicities, and 274 languages. The Brazilian Institute of Geography and Statistics (IBGE) notes that 83% of indigenous people aged over ten years old receive the minimum wage or less. Although there are indigenous populations in all five regions of Brazil, the Northern Region has the greatest concentration with 342,800 indigenous inhabitants occupying 12.5% of the Brazilian territory (IBGE,

2012a, 2012b; Brasil 2015). As a result, Brazil is often considered to be one of the most socio-culturally diverse countries on the planet given that, by way of comparison, there are only 140 indigenous languages in the whole of the European continent (Fellet, 2016).

In terms of distribution and supply of medically trained health professionals, Brazil underperforms compared to international standards, with only 1.8 doctors per 1,000 inhabitants: Canada has 2.0, the UK 2.7, Portugal 3.9, and Spain 4.0 doctors per 1,000 inhabitants (OMS, 2010). By comparison, the Amazon region has the lowest concentration of doctors, with only 0.98 doctors per 1,000 inhabitants.

The Brazilian Amazon (see Figure 2.1) is actually composed of nine States that border Peru, Bolivia, Colombia, Guiana, and Venezuela. There have been a multitude of different governments and administrative bodies overseeing the organization and management of the Brazilian Amazon. During the military dictatorship, between 1964 and 1985, development projects resulted in significant environmental and social transformation, such as the construction of roads, hydroelectric plants, agrarian reform, mining, and urbanization. During the democratic transition, the Amazon region was characterized by social inclusion projects that contrasted. and often conflicted, with that local development, agribusiness, and hydroelectric agenda (Baines, 2017; Brasil, 2008).

In this chapter, we will draw mostly on the experience of the State of Amazonas because it has the lowest rate of deforestation and the highest number of indigenous reserves and nature reserves. In addition, access to municipalities in the interior of the State of Amazonas is almost entirely via the rivers and tributaries,

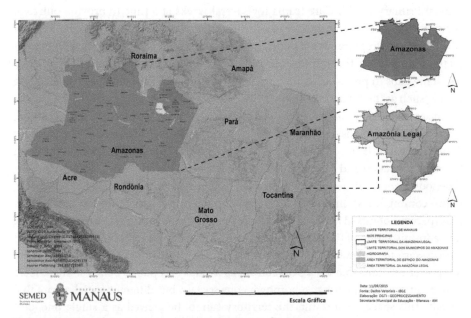

Figure 2.1 Map of the Amazon showing the State of Amazonas.

posing unique challenges. Rivers, streams, and lakes form the fluvial network, and there are enormous distances between municipalities and an extremely low population density (2.23 inhabitants per km^2). The State of Amazonas corresponds to 18.4% of the entire national territory (IBGE, 2014) and borders Venezuela, Colombia, and Peru.

2.3 Primary care, public health, and the 'fluid territory'

Healthcare public health in the State of Amazonas is supported by a variety of health-care policies that complement primary care in an approach that is intersectoral and integrated. For example, the Healthy School Programme is a government initiative that supports improvements in the health of children between the ages of two and six years by linking school attendance to vaccination completion rates and nutritional surveillance. The Street Consultation Programme seeks to improve access to population groups that are living in precarious or vulnerable conditions, through multidisciplinary health teams. The Family Health Support Teams are composed of physiotherapists, pharmacists, nutritionists, psychologists, and social workers and provide multidisciplinary professional advice in complex clinical cases. These teams ensure collaborative design of individual therapeutic care plans and support ESF teams to develop comprehensive strategies for the prevention and promotion of health in the community. The Fluvial Primary Health Care Units are custom-made boats with the necessary equipment, environment, and accommodation to transport Fluvial Primary Health Care teams for several weeks at a time to provide outreach services that meet the healthcare needs of remote fluvial communities. Finally, the More Doctors Programme is a policy created by interministerial decree with the objective of improving the training, recruitment, and retention of primary care doctors, to fill the gaps in provision in the areas of greatest social inequality and challenging access, such as the Amazon region.

The entire territory of the Amazon region directly reflects environmental, cultural, and ethnic dimensions and the historical processes of land occupation. The territory is not static, but is in constant movement and transformation, and this impacts on the administration and development of public policies. Occupying this space are indigenous people, riverside communities, mineworkers, quilombolas (indigenous negro communities), internally displaced populations, settlers, migrants, and caboclos (persons of mixed heritage)—all actors that influence and effect the organization and administration of the space. According to the geographer Becker (2005, 2010), it is necessary to understand the territories, and their transformations, because there are power relations that exist between social groups and public policies. There is no single, unique State, neither a homogeneous society, but different social actors that dispute this space. As a result, the territory cannot be viewed as a single one, or a homogeneous one, and is marked by contrasts that have constructed and formed the social, political, and economic histories.

Within this perspective, the territory is a geographic space with multiple social and power relations that requires delicate and careful negotiation. The sheer magnitude of the fluvial network mandates a consideration of healthcare public health as a fluid entity. The cycle of the 'waters' has four distinct phases: the dry period, the flooded period, and the in-between phases of ebbing and flowing. All these impact on the lives of the local populations and, as a result, the work of the primary care teams. In the State of Amazonas, for example, houses are built on stilts or, in some cases, are even built to float, enabling them to be moved in times of the greatest flooding (see Figures 2.2 and 2.3).

Riverside communities construct their homes and pursue their lives within the cycles of the rivers. Their homes are located alongside the rivers, and they move only by using the rivers. In the dry periods, communities can become isolated, and the transportation of people and goods becomes complicated, although the exposed land is used productively for goat herding and cultivation of fruits and vegetables. In the flooded season, transportation is facilitated but the cultivated land becomes flooded. Healthcare public health needs to be constructed within this fluid dynamic, and primary care, healthcare networks, and care pathways need to accommodate the shifting realities. The movements and shifting flows follow their own logic and do not always adhere to the rigidities of public policies.

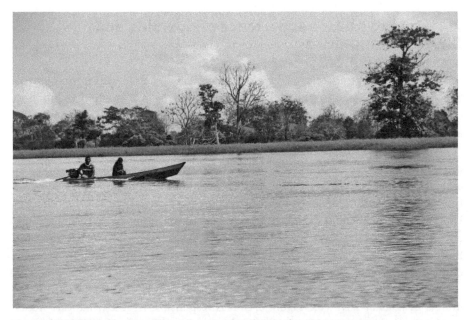

Figure 2.2 A typical boat used to transport families in the Amazon region.
Photo: Reproduced courtesy of Julio Cesar Schweickardt

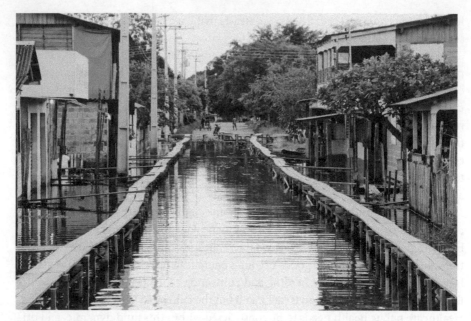

Figure 2.3 Riverside communities constructed on stilts in the Borba Municipality, State of Amazonas.
Photo: Reproduced courtesy of Nicolas Esteban Heufemann

2.4 The healthcare experience of riverside and fluvial communities

In the past, ambulatory care was provided to riverside communities through the transport of healthcare teams by boat, and care was delivered in schools, churches, or peoples' homes. These teams were organized on a 'campaign' basis—periodically, and usually during immunization campaigns or outbreaks such as malaria and other endemic infections. In order to provide the type of fundamental primary health-care as established in the ministerial decrees and health policies of the PNAB, several adaptations were necessary to take into account this dynamic context. In 2011, the Ministry of Health financed the construction of 64 Fluvial Primary Health Care Units (UBSFs) that could journey the entire lengths of the rivers, according to the ebbs and flows of the water levels, and provide increased access to healthcare for these populations and meet the needs of the riverside communities of the nine States of the Amazon region.

The UBSF Igaracu, in the Municipality of Borba, was the first boat to be inaugurated, in January 2013 (see Figure 2.4). It is responsible for the healthcare needs of 12,000 inhabitants in 230 communities in the Rio Madeira. The UBSF also has smaller boats that can be launched in narrower rivers to reach various communities. The UBSF Igaracu is 24 metres in length and has two floors. The lower floor is for

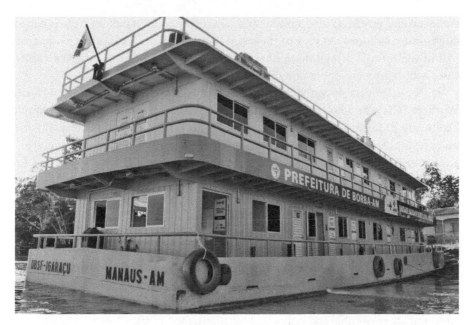

Figure 2.4 Fluvial Primary Care Unit, UBSF Igaracu, in the Barba Municipality, State of Amazonas.

Photo: Reproduced courtesy of Nicolas Esteban Heufemann

ambulatory care and has a doctors' consultation room, a nursing area, a dentistry, a pharmacy, a treatment room for minor operations and dressing changes, and a room for immunizations, materials, and sterilization. The upper floor comprises accommodation for the crew and the health professionals, all of whom can spend up to 20 days on board.

Since 2012, the PNAB has decreed that each UBSF should be composed of a nurse, doctor, nurse technician, laboratory technician, dentist, and dental technician. The teams actually deliver the majority of their care in primary care units within the specific communities that can be reached via the rivers and streams, whilst the more distant communities are reached and attended to on the boats themselves. In the Amazon region, the time taken to travel between communities is a more common measure than the physical distance itself. The time taken to travel between communities is also highly variable as a function of the dry and flooded seasons. The distances in the dry season are much greater; in the flooded season, the time taken to travel is less due to the number of shortcuts that can be found.

The teams are expected to provide consultations on the boats for at least 14 days per month, eight hours per day, with two days allowed for continuing education, maintaining records, data management, and planning. For communities that are more distant, the teams are expected to organize their journeys in such a way that all communities are reached at least once every 60 days, in order to meet the requirements of antenatal and postnatal care, growth and development in infants, and management of chronic conditions. As part of their day-to-day activities, referrals are organized within the team and multidisciplinary discussions are held over complex clinical cases, which promotes the comprehensive approach to clinical care.

In the intervals between visits, support is provided by the Community Health Workers (CHWs) who, although minimally trained in some simple, common healthcare problems, serve as the critical link between the community, the primary healthcare team and health professionals, and municipality management and administration. Through the ESF, there are now over 250,000 CHWs across the entire country, supporting ESF primary care teams through home visits, outreach activity, community development, and social support (Macinko & Harris, 2015). In the case of fluvial communities, CHWs and nurse technicians are also expected to live within the riverside communities and to work 40 hours per week (Brasil, 2012, 2017).

The CHWs perform an essential function in health promotion and illness prevention, by providing health literacy and education programmes and well-being activities such as community groups, 'knit and natter' groups, and counselling services. Amongst other essential and important functions, the CHWs:

(a) register all the inhabitants of the micro-territory that they are responsible for and maintain all health records;
(b) signpost families with respect to available healthcare services;
(c) implement programmed activities to manage spontaneous demand; and
(d) monitor, through regular home visits, all families that are within their areas of responsibility.

Home visits by CHWs are scheduled with the team and take into account risk and vulnerability factors, such that families with the greatest need can be visited more frequently, whilst maintaining a minimum of one home visit per month for all households in each micro-territory that that they are responsible for. This provides a safety net for the entire community, and not just those targeted based on arbitrary socio-demographic characteristics.

2.5 Indigenous health policy

There are around one million indigenous people living in Brazil (IBGE, 2010). The State of Amazonas has the largest concentration of indigenous people in Brazil (17%). The largest ethnic group is the Tikuna, with 30,000 inhabitants. Four of the fifteen largest indigenous population groups are in the State of Amazonas: the Yanomami (who also live in the State of Roraima), the Satere–Mawe, the Mundurucu, and the Mura. Indigenous populations are a minority within Brazilian society, and 'the majority of the indigenous population are micro-societies' (Langdon, 2004, p. 15).

The 1988 Brazilian Constitution recognizes the multicultural character of Brazilian society, in that public policy is grounded in the principle of tolerance in all dimensions. From this point of departure, the Brazilian government organized a subsystem for health that is uniquely different for the indigenous population that is particularly at great risk and vulnerable. The legislation that addresses the indigenous population and its access to healthcare speaks as much to the use and practice of western medicine and techniques as it does to the practices and traditions of indigenous medicine. The policy notes that 'primary care delivered through health units should be considered as complimentary to, not substituting of, traditional practices and there is an explicit concern to ensure that health protection and promotion through official routes are delivered alongside diverse forms of indigenous practice of self-care' (Langdon, 2004, p. 37).

The successful establishment and recognition of the rights of the indigenous population were achieved through a long-running social movement in Brazil. The degree of autonomy and self-identification affects decisions that indigenous people make over their lives and livelihoods, including the use of natural resources, cultural resources, such as language and social organization, educational and administrative systems, and the valuing and strengthening of local knowledge systems (Little, 2002).

The healthcare system for indigenous health is organized into 34 Special Indigenous Sanitary Districts (DSEIs) across the whole country and reflects the SUS as a whole in that it is divided into levels of technological density with health promotion, protection, and rehabilitation integrated and equitably provided for all service users. The Special Secretariat for Indigenous Health (SESAI) is linked to the Ministry of Health and is responsible for the care of all indigenous people that is delivered through the DSEIs. DSEIs are organized according to the geographical location of indigenous communities, and these do not necessarily reflect geopolitical boundaries of States or Municipalities. According to the National Policy for Healthcare of Indigenous People, the 34 DSEIs must be structured to provide simple ambulatory care in its Central Pole, with medium and high complexity clinical care the responsibility of local hospitals. The significance of this is that there is a subsystem within the SUS, reliant on its own funding base and processes for financing care (Brasil, 2002). Referral for hospital care is via a referral system at the Central Pole to the Centre for Indigenous Health (CASAI), based either in the main municipal or State headquarters, or directly to the local hospitals.

The establishment of the DSEI is considered a significant policy advance, but it is still fraught with a variety of tensions. In the SUS, resources for primary care are transferred from the federal government on a per capita basis. Resources for primary care are also transferred for each DSEI for the indigenous population in the same locality. Finally, both the DSEI and the municipality can provide primary care services to indigenous people, within the primary care systems or within the secondary and tertiary care levels, given that the system is considered to be universal.

The structure and organization of indigenous population health is the result of a lengthy political battle by their leaders and representatives (CIMI, 2013), motivated by the pursuit of the integrity, respect, and autonomy of indigenous cultures. This provides an example of how national policies have needed to adapt to the specificities of local realities and cultures. The major challenge in this subsystem is how to ensure a dialogue between the traditions of indigenous medicine and those of contemporary medicine. For this, it has been necessary to guarantee ongoing and continuous professional development for health professionals that service different ethnic groups, to provide a service that is integrated and equitable.

The central features of healthcare public health for indigenous populations are health promotion and strategic programmes for the prevention and control of disease. As such, indigenous health services mirror those of the PNAB within the logic of strategic programmes and a strong focus on teams living and working within the territory and with the necessary infrastructure to guarantee integrated care (Pontes et al., 2015). This 'territorialization' is a radical departure from how healthcare services were previously delivered mostly through campaign-based programmes.

The healthcare services are composed of Village Health Posts, staffed by Indigenous Health Agents (AIS) and nurse technicians who are generally themselves of an indigenous ethnicity. Being from the indigenous community, they understand the reality of the service users and contribute significantly to the exchange of traditional practices with biomedical knowledge, presenting and contextualizing this for the Indigenous Health Team (EMSI). An example of the interaction between contemporary and traditional knowledge in primary care is the production of intercultural care. Health professionals work closely with the AISs to translate contemporary medical terminologies into concepts compatible with indigenous knowledge bases. and often will liaise with traditional birth attendants to share care and management. In many cases, doctors (who until late 2018 were predominantly of Cuban origin as a result of the More Doctors Programme) will prescribe contemporary biomedical treatments alongside the use of traditional medicines, herbs, and teas and the practices of traditional soothsayers, quacks, indigenous priests, and religious leaders (Erthal, 2001). In this sense, health professionals, trained in the biomedical tradition, are required to constantly encounter this intercultural dialogue. Healthcare public health of indigenous populations is extremely complex due to the geographical diversity of the territory, as well as the peculiarities of the relationships within communities. Their culture and ways of life are particularly unique.

Of the 28 communities covered by the Betania Indigenous Health Hub, the majority,—a population of around 4,800 people—inhabit the length of the River Ica, and depend on fishing, extractive industries, and farming. In addition to the extreme poverty, there are immense distances to the primary healthcare services and more sophisticated levels of healthcare. As a result, these communities are reached only once per month, and sometimes even less frequently depending on whether the boats, fuel, and healthcare teams are available. Doctors are often unavailable and teams might be dispatched without them. Given that the majority of doctors that work within the indigenous healthcare system are not in fact Brazilian, it has been extremely challenging to retain doctors in the EMSI, particularly in those areas more distant from regional capitals. The majority of the doctors have been recruited through the More Doctors Programme and are, therefore, only able to provide services for 15 days out of every month at a time. Nonetheless, when in attendance, they will develop a wide range of health promotion activities within the Primary Care Health Unit, and provide home visits in urgent cases or where the service user has difficulty travelling. This often entails working 24-hour shifts, including for urgent cases and obstetric care, and will often occur in their own place of residence.

In the communities where indigenous languages are spoken, AISs also serve as interpreters, facilitating the interaction between patient, relatives, and the team. They have a very important role in the connection between the service and the population within their territory and area of responsibility, and are also involved in the development of unique activities. As cultural translators, they can produce cultural hybridization between traditional and biomedical knowledge bases (Brasil, 2002). The AISs also play an important active role in promoting social and community participation in the construction and design of healthcare services suitable for the needs of the local population.

This role as cultural translator has contributed not only to an improved understanding of medical issues by the indigenous populations, but also a mediation between cultural concepts present in these collocated spaces of 'interculturality'. In the last few decades, this concept of interculturality in health (or intercultural health) has been used to designate those activities and policies that seek to incorporate the culture of the patient into healthcare (Yajahuanca et al., 2015). Interculturality brings an array of symbolic challenges and power relations that are in themselves asymmetrical, and can represent a method for managing ethnic and cultural differences (Ferreira, 2015; WIIO, 2017). However, discursive and interpretive questions such as these need to be presented, elaborated, and understood. This question of interculturality in healthcare, arrived at from the contrasting spaces of traditional and contemporary perspectives, is more about a relationship of respect and tolerance, education and development on the part of the health professionals, quacks, priests, and soothsayers than the incorporation of particular techniques and practices.

The work of the AISs—that on a daily basis is limited by physical, technological, and cognitive constraints—produces results and impact that are relevant for health and health outcomes. However, this work also potentiates health professionals, overcoming limitations that are often present in the professional development of health workers in other settings (Kadri et al., 2017).

2.6 Final considerations

In this chapter, we have reviewed the types of healthcare services and professionals available across the Amazon region—a region characterized by extreme distance, geography, and cultural diversity. The characteristics of the healthcare territory have necessitated different types of delivery models, adapted best practice, and availability of professionals across a wide spectrum of disciplines and geographies. Healthcare public health is most effective when it reflects the realities of the local population and their ways of life in extreme environments. Fluid territories have been used to adapt to the reality of dry and flooded seasons. Intercultural health has led to the co-production of cultural practices, whether biomedical or traditional, and their absorption into healthcare delivery. Identity and culture are potent in how knowledge is produced and shared in this region. The model of indigenous healthcare seeks to integrate traditional and biomedical systems in the production of health promotion and protection activities. Finally, clinical and cultural competency are therefore essential to develop appropriate models of healthcare public health in the Amazon region.

Abbreviations

AIS Agente Indígena de Saúde, Indigenous Health Agent
DSEI Distrito Sanitario Especiais Indigiena, Special Indigenous Sanitary Districts
EMSI Equipe Multiprofissional de Saúde Indígena, Indigenous Health Team
ESF Estrategia Saude da Familia, Family Health Strategy
IBGE Instituto Brasileiro de Geografia e Estatistica, Brazilian Institute of Geography and
    Statistics
PNAB Programa National de Atencao Basica, National Primary Care Programme
PSF Programa Saude da Familia, Family Health Programme
SUS Sistema Unico de Saude, Unified Health System
UBSF Unidade Basica de Saude Fluvial, Riverside Basic Health Unit

References

Aquino, R., Medina, M.G., Nunes, C.A., & Sousa, M.F. (2014). Estratégia Saúde da Família e Reordenamento do sistema de serviços de saúde. In: J. Paim & N. Almeida Filho (eds) *Saúde Coletiva: Teoria e Prática*. Rio de Janeiro: Medbook, pp. 353–371.

Aquino, R., Medina, M.G., Vilasbôas, A.L.Q., & Barreto, M.L. (2009). Programa de saúde da família: análise de sua implantação no Brasil. In: L.R. Silva L.R (ed.) *Diagnóstico em Pediatria*. Rio de Janeiro: Guanabara Koogan, pp. 1031–1040.

Baines, S. (2017). Projetos de desenvolvimento na Amazônia e as estratégias de grandes empresas. *Revista sobre acesso à justiça e direitos nas Américas, Brasília*, 1(1), 297–314.

Becker, B. (2005). Geopolítica da Amazônia. *Estudos Avançados, São Paulo*, 19(53), 71–86.

Becker, B. (2010). Novas territorialidades na Amazônia: desafio às políticas públicas. *Bol Mus Para Emílio Goeldi Ciênc Hum, Belém*, 5(1), 17–23.

Brasil (Ministério da Saúde). (2002). *Política Nacional de Atenção à Saúde dos Povos Indígenas*. Brasília: Fundação Nacional de Saúde.

Brasil (Governo Federal). (2008). *Plano Amazônia Sustentável: diretrizes para o desenvolvimento sustentável da Amazônia Brasileira*. Brasília: MMA.

Brasil (Ministério da Saúde). (2012). *Política Nacional de Atenção Básica*. Brasília: Ministério da Saúde.

Brasil (Governo Federal). (2015). *Populações Indígenas do Brasil*. Brasília: Secretaria Especial de Saúde Indígena. Available at: http://www.brasil.gov.br/governo/2015/04/populacao-indigena-no-brasil-e-de-896-9-mil [accessed 20 August 2015].

Brasil (Ministério da Saúde). (2017). *Portaria 2436, de 21 de setembro de 2017. Aprova a Política Nacional de Atenção Básica no âmbito do SUS*. Brasília, DF: Ministério da Saúde. Available at:: http://www.brasilsus.com.br/index.php/legislacoes/gabinete-do-ministro/16247 [accessed 5 December 2018].

Conselho Indigenista Missionário (CIMI). (2013). *A Política de Atenção à Saúde Indígena no Brasil. Breve recuperação histórica sobre a política de assistência à saúde nas comunidades indígenas*. Brasil: CNBB.

Erthal, R.M.C. (2001). O suicídio Ticuna no Alto Solimões: uma expressão de conflitos. *Cad Saúde Pública* 17, 299–311.

Fellet, J. (2016). 'Dia do Índio': estudo revela 305 etnias e 274 línguas entre povos indígenas do Brasil. BBC News Brasil. Available at: https://www.bbc.com/portuguese/brasil-36682290 [accessed 29 December 2018].

Ferreira, L.O. (2015). Interculturalidade e saúde indígena no contexto das políticas públicas brasileiras. In: E.J. Langdon & M.D. Cardoso (eds) *Saúde indígena: políticas comparadas na América Latina*. Florianópolis: Editora UFSC.

Hone, T., et al. (2017). Association between expansion of primary healthcare and racial inequalities in mortality amenable to primary care in Brazil: a national longitudinal analysis. *PLOS Med*, 4(5), e1002306.

Instituto Brasileiro de Geografia e Estatística (IBGE). (2012a). *Censo demográfico 2010. Características gerais dos indígenas. Resultados do universo*. Rio de Janeiro: IBGE. Available at: http://www.ibge.gov.br/estadosat/perfil.php?sigla=am [accessed 4 September 2015].

Instituto Brasileiro de Geografia e Estatística (IBGE). (2012b). *Censo demografico indígena 2012*. Available at: https://agenciadenoticias.ibge.gov.br/agencia-sala-de-imprensa/2013-agencia-de-noticias/releases/14262-asi-censo-2010-populacao-indigena-e-de-8969-mil-tem-305-etnias-e-fala-274-idiomas [accessed29 December 2018].

Kadri, M.R., Schweickardt, J.C., & Lima, R.T.S. (2017). *Território Líquido: A Unidade Básica de Saúde Fluvial 'Igaraçu'. Anais do VIII Simpósio Nacional de Geografia da Saúde, Dourados, MS, 27 de junho a 01 de julho de 2017*. Dourados, MS: UFGD/ GESF.

Langdon, E.J. (2004). Uma avaliação crítica da atenção diferenciada e a colaboração entre antropologia e profissionais de saúde. In: E.J. & L. Garnelo (eds) *Saúde dos Povos Indígenas: reflexões sobre antropologia participativa*. Rio de Janeiro: Contra Capa; ABA.

Lima, R.T.S., Simões, A.L., Heufemann, N.E., & Alves, V.P. (2016). Saúde sobre as águas: o caso da Unidade Básica de Saúde Fluvial. In: R.B. Ceccim, J.A. Kreutz, J.D.P. Campos, F.S. Culau, L.A.F. Wottrich, & L.L. Kessler (eds) *Intensidade na atenção básica: prospecção de experiências 'informes' e pesquisa-formação*. Porto Alegre: Rede Unida, pp. 269–293.

Little, P. (2002). Etnodesenvolvimento local: autonomia cultural na era do neoliberalismo global. *Tellus*, 3, 33–52.

Macinko, J., et al. (2010). Major expansion of primary care in Brazil linked to decline in unnecessary hospitalization. *Health Aff*, 29 (12), 2149–2160.

Macinko, J. & Harris, M. (2015). Brazil's family health strategy—delivering community-based primary care in a universal health system. *New Engl J Med*, 372(23), 2177–2181.

Organização Mundial da Saúde (OMS). (2010). *Increasing Access to Health Workers in Remote and Rural Areas through Improved Retention: Global Recommendations*. Geneva: OMS.

Paim, J. (2015). *O que é o SUS*. Rio de Janeiro: Ed. Fiocruz.

Pontes, A.L.M., Rego, S., & Garnelo, L. (2015). O modelo de atenção diferenciada nos Distritos Sanitários Especiais Indígenas: reflexões a partir do Alto Rio Negro/AM, Brasil. *Ciência e Saúde Coletiva*, 20(10), 3199–3210.

Rasella, D., Harhay, M.O., Pamponet, M.L., Aquino, R., & Barreto, M.L. (2014). Impact of primary health care on mortality from heart and cerebrovascular diseases in Brazil: a nationwide analysis of longitudinal data. *BMJ (Clin Res)*, 349(5), 4014.

Rasella, D., Aquino, R., & Barreto, M.L. (2010). Reducing childhood mortality from diarrhea and lower respiratory tract infections in Brazil. *Pediatrics*, 126(3), e534–540.

Rocha, R. & Soares, R.R. (2010). Evaluating the impact of community-based health interventions: evidence from Brazil's family health program. *Health Econ*, 158, 126–158.

Starfield B. (2002). Atenção primária de saúde: equilíbrio entre necessidades de saúde, serviços e tecnologia. Brasilia: Unesco, Ministério da Saúde.

World Bank. (2019). GINI Index (World Bank Estimate). Washington, DC: World Bank. Available at: https://data.worldbank.org/indicator/SI.POV.GINI?locations=BR [accessed 16 July 2019].

World Health Organization & Pan American Health Organization. (2017). Policy on ethnicity and health, 25–29 September 2017. Washington, DC: Pan American Health Organization.

Yajahuanca, R.A., Diniz, C.S.G., & Cabral, C.S. (2015). É preciso 'ikarar os kutipados': interculturalidade e assistência à saúde na Amazônia Peruana. *Ciênc Saúde Coletiva*, Rio de Janeiro, 20(9), 2837–2846.

3
Promoting equity through health services

Bo Burström

3.1 Introduction

This chapter discusses the role of health services in reducing inequalities and promoting equity in access to care among vulnerable and underserved groups. The underlying assumptions for the chapter are illustrated in Figure 3.1. The unequal distribution of the determinants of health causes inequalities in health status. Poor health status translates into a perceived need of care, which results in a demand for, and consumption of, healthcare (Burström, 2009). Ideally, the care and treatment obtained leads to improved health outcomes.

The degree to which symptoms of poor health status are perceived as a need of care varies between different groups, and may be related to different factors, including the level of health literacy of the individual. Health literacy has been defined as 'the degree to which individuals have the capacity to obtain, process, and understand basic health information and services needed to make appropriate health decisions' (Ratzan & Parker, 2000). Health literacy also plays a role in negotiating care, and in how patients convey their problem to a healthcare provider (Adams et al., 2009), which in turn may impact on what treatment they receive.

In the chain of events described in Figure 3.1, inequalities between socioeconomic groups may arise at many of the steps (Gulliford, 2003). People with a low level of health literacy may seek healthcare later than those with a high level of health literacy. When translating need into demand for healthcare services, other factors such as geographic and economic access to care may intervene to facilitate or hinder this. This step may also be affected by previous experiences of care and by cultural factors. Then, the way in which the individual presents his or her symptoms and communicates with the healthcare provider will be important for being properly understood and getting the right care and treatment for the health condition. Here again, health literacy may play an important role: a good knowledge of both the language and the relevant concepts will help the individual to communicate with the care provider; whilst on the other hand, a recent immigrant to a country may lack this knowledge, which may hinder proper understanding and treatment. Whether the treatment and consumption of care leads to an improved health outcome also depends on the quality of the care provided, which may vary for different patients.

Bo Burström, *Promoting equity through health services* In: *Healthcare Public Health*. Edited by: Martin Gulliford and Edmund Jessop, Oxford University Press (2020). © Oxford University Press. DOI: 10.1093/oso/9780198837206.003.0003.

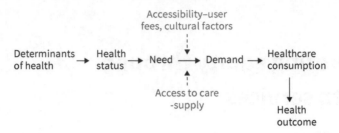

Figure 3.1 Inequalities in health and healthcare.

Reproduced with permission from Burström B. 'Market-oriented, demand-driven health care reforms and equity in health and health care utilization in Sweden.' *International Journal of Health Services.* Volume 39, Issue 2, pp. 271–85. Copyright © 2009 Sage Publications.

There are several examples of inequalities arising between different groups in the steps just described. For instance, the mortality among people with chronic heart failure differs between those with high and low health literacy, even when adjusted for disease staging and biomedical parameters (Peterson et al., 2011). In Sweden, although poorly educated women have a lower incidence rate of breast cancer, they have a higher breast cancer mortality rate than well-educated women (Beiki et al., 2012). Women with the highest level of education have 20–30% higher incidence but 30–40% lower case fatality rates compared with women with the lowest level of education, suggesting that poorly educated women do not attend breast cancer screening or do not adhere to the recommended treatment to the same extent as well-educated women (Beiki et al., 2012).

International studies show that proximity to healthcare facilities increases the likelihood of seeking care, and that low-income earners have a higher likelihood, compared to high-income earners, of abstaining from seeking care for economic reasons, despite perceiving a need (Corscadden et al., 2018). In a study based on secondary analysis of the 2016 Commonwealth Fund International Health Policy Survey of Adults in 11 countries (Australia, Canada, France, Germany, Norway, the Netherlands, New Zealand, Sweden, Switzerland, the UK, and the USA), the adjusted odds ratio among low-income earners of abstaining from care across countries was 1.22 to 3.32 (Corscadden et al., 2018).

Some groups of patients may have higher mortality rates for the same disease and receive care of lower quality than other groups, as illustrated by a study of mortality and quality indicators of treatment among people with and without a previous inpatient episode for psychiatric disease (Björkenstam et al., 2012). People with a history of psychiatric disease had higher rates of death from conditions considered amenable to intervention by the health service (that is, avoidable mortality). Among people admitted for myocardial infarction, the 28-day case death rate was higher among those previously admitted for psychiatric inpatient care than among other people: 53.5 (42.0–65.0) among women admitted for schizophrenia compared to 26.5 (25.7–27.3) among other women. Among people with diabetes, those previously admitted for schizophrenia had lower rates (40.9: 36.8–45.1) than other women (56.1: 55.7–56.2) of prescriptions for blood lipid lowering statins, as secondary prevention for their health condition (Björkenstam et al., 2012).

Finally, there may be socioeconomic differences in the cost of care in the last year of life, suggesting differential treatment and care (Hanratty et al., 2007). A study on Swedish data found that public health spending on care in the last year of life was higher among high-income groups than among low-income groups. Median per capita expenditure was 55,417 Swedish Kronor (SEK) (US$ 7,542) in the lowest income group and SEK 94,678 (US$ 12,887) in the highest income group. The significant difference remained even after adjusting for age, sex, healthcare utilization, and major diagnostic groups (Hanratty et al., 2007).

3.2 Market-oriented reforms, access to healthcare, and how people seek and receive care: an example from Sweden

Sweden has a tax-funded, largely publicly provided healthcare system. The responsibility for healthcare—with collecting taxes and funding the greatest part of the costs—lies at regional/county council level. Since the 1980s, there have been publicly funded initiatives to increase the marketization and privatization of healthcare provision (Svallfors & Tyllström, 2018). Attempts have also been made to increase the role of primary care and access. Some 15–17% of doctors in Sweden work in primary care (Isaksson et al., 2016).

In 2010, a national law was enacted to allow the free establishment of privately operated primary care clinics funded by the county council, and the free choice of primary care provider (with payment to the provider linked to the individual). The reform was intended to increase access to primary care, and did result in 285 new primary care clinics, 95% of which are operating at a profit (Isaksson et al., 2016). There was a corresponding increase in the number of patient visits; however, this increase was observed mainly among people with lesser needs (Agerholm et al., 2015; Riksrevisionen [National Audit Office], 2014).

At the same time, the reform allowing the freedom of where to establish new clinics limited the ability of the county councils to direct new, privately provided services to where the need was greatest. As a consequence, the number of clinics increased mainly in affluent urban areas in bigger cities, and there was no impact (or in some cases, actually a deterioration of access to care) in rural areas and disadvantaged areas in cities (Riksrevisionen [National Audit Office], 2014; Isaksson, 2016; Dahlgren, 2018).

A parallel development took place in the social care of older people. Long-term residential care and home care of older people is the responsibility of social services at local (municipal) level. In 2009, similar reform allowed for the choice and expansion of private providers in residential care and home care of older people. A government investigation reported, in 2016, that the reform regarding choice in primary care and social care actually counteracted coordination and integration of care among older people with complex health and social care needs, and proposed that older people with such needs should be exempted from the reform (Regeringen [Government of Sweden], 2016).

3.3 Changes in resource allocation and in the reimbursement system in primary care

Before primary care reform, Stockholm County Council had used a need-based system for resource allocation in primary care (Burström et al., 2017a), based primarily on weighted capitation (by sociodemographic characteristics of the population in the catchment area, known to be related to ill health and need of care). The system redistributed quite substantial funds according to need. The area with the highest-weighted capitation was estimated to receive one and a half to two times more funds compared to the average for the whole county council. This system remained in place up until 2008, when it was exchanged for another system based on fee-for-service and unweighted capitation. The change meant that primary care clinics in more disadvantaged areas lost the substantial extra resources they had previously received and had to reduce their staff numbers.

The change coincided with the implementation of the reform in primary care, which was launched earlier (2008) in Stockholm County Council than in the rest of the country (2010). The emphasis in the new reimbursement system was on fee-for-service (60% of reimbursement was based on the number of visits), and the capitation part (40% of the reimbursement) was not weighted by need or for socioeconomic factors. This meant that the clinic had to produce a greater number of visits in order to make up for the lost income from weighted capitation. The new reimbursement system incentivized short visits, and chronic patients with complex problems and requiring longer visits were deprioritized. Analyses have shown that the increase in visits following the reform and change in reimbursement was greater among people with a higher income and higher level of education, than among less well-educated people with greater needs (Agerholm et al., 2015; Burström et al., 2017a)

Reimbursement systems are important as they may impact on how doctors work and how healthcare services are operated, and which patients are prioritized. In primary care, reimbursement may be based on capitation, fee-for-service, or meeting certain performance indicator goals. The different reimbursement systems may operate in different ways—to benefit (or not) the provision of care to people with greater needs. For instance, if the capitation is the same for all and not weighted to take into account socioeconomic differences in health and healthcare needs in the population, it will give more resources (in relative terms) to areas with lesser needs (Burström et al., 2017a).

In spite of the importance of reimbursement systems, and their impact on equity in the provision of healthcare services and prioritization of patients, few studies have specifically investigated the aspect of equity. However, in a recent review of studies (Tao et al., 2016), no firm conclusions could be drawn regarding the equity impact of a particular reimbursement system, as the impact may differ between different diseases, and may be dependent on the type of healthcare system and on the impact of other policy aspects.

3.4 What could be done to reduce inequalities in healthcare?

3.4.1 Resource allocation

One important starting point when considering how to reduce inequalities in healthcare is that healthcare should be provided according to need of care. This is often stated in the health policy documents of different countries, and also implies that resources for healthcare should be distributed by need. The operationalization and measurement of need differs, but often takes into account disease status and health status (Carr–Hill et al., 1990; Gravelle et al., 2003).

In view of the greater burden of disease and poorer health among lower socioeconomic groups, the need of care is greater amongst these groups than amongst higher socioeconomic groups. Hence, lower socioeconomic groups should receive more resources, and areas where a greater proportion of the population are poorly educated or have other characteristics which indicate a greater need of care should receive more healthcare resources. Such need-based allocation of resources is practiced in the UK (NHS, 2018) and was previously used in parts of Sweden (Diderichsen et al., 1997).

Although it may be difficult to evaluate the impact of need-based resource allocation on health indicators, a study by Barr et al. (2014) showed a more rapid decline of mortality amenable to healthcare in areas receiving more resources, compared to areas not receiving extra resources. Between 2001 and 2011, the increase in NHS resources to deprived areas accounted for a reduction in the gap between deprived and affluent areas in male mortality amenable to healthcare of 35 deaths per 100,000 population (95% confidence interval: 27–42) and, in female mortality, of 16 deaths per 100,000 (95% confidence interval: 10–21) (Barr et al., 2014).

3.4.2 Provision of services

Although rates of disease and disability are higher in disadvantaged areas than in other areas, people may not seek care to match their needs. Other types of outreach activities may be needed, in order for them to make contact with appropriate healthcare services (Morgan, 2003). In the provision of healthcare services, the different needs and different patterns of health-seeking behaviours of different population groups should be taken into consideration. For instance, in delivering primary care to the population in disadvantaged areas, it might be important not only to deal with patients who seek care at the clinic but also to consider alternative ways, such as outreach activities, of reaching those people with unmet needs.

In Stockholm County Council, some primary care clinics in disadvantaged areas receive extra funds for community-oriented health promotion and disease prevention activities, in collaboration with other local actors (Fritzell et al., 2016). Some clinics perform 'Health days' in the local area. On these occasions, staff from the clinic meet with local residents, outside the clinic. Staff take measurements of blood glucose level and blood pressure, provide information about smoking cessation services, discuss the importance of physical activity and good dietary habits, and advise residents about the primary care clinic. These meetings with residents have resulted in the detection of new cases of diabetes and hypertension, and have encouraged people who previously had no contact with the clinic to visit and become regular patients. This way of working is appreciated by the residents (Fritzell et al., 2016).

The prevalence of diabetes is high in some disadvantaged areas in greater Stockholm (Tao et al., 2015). These patients need regular check-up and management, and also retinal examinations by eye specialists. Normally, these examinations take place at the specialist eye hospital in the centre of the city, but attendance rates have been lower for patients from disadvantaged area, who have not travelled there. In some areas, the primary care clinic has therefore collaborated with the specialist eye hospital to perform such examinations locally, in order to increase the rate of eye examinations (Fritzell et al., 2016).

Staff from primary care clinics, recognizing that their patients are sedentary and need more physical exercise, have organized regular walking groups, for those patients who want to participate. Other examples of outreach activities include the formation of social support groups for people of working age who, for health reasons, are outside the labour market (Fritzell et al., 2016).

3.4.3 Practicing proportionate universalism: extended postnatal home visiting in a disadvantaged area

Maternal and child health services have a long tradition and reach almost the entire population in Sweden. These services are well known and respected, and contribute to good maternal and child health. There is an extensive schedule of visits to nurses and doctors. Mothers are called to the clinic for monitoring throughout the pregnancy, and from childbirth until the child turns six years of age. The scheme includes one home visit, offered to all parents when their child is about two weeks old.

However, the need of care varies between different groups in the population, and is greater in some disadvantaged areas. The population in one residential area (Rinkeby) in a Stockholm municipality includes a large proportion of recent immigrants. Unemployment is high in the area, and the majority of families are on a low income or social assistance. Child health is less good than in other areas, and social services are involved with more families here than in other areas (Burström et al., 2017b).

Studies from the USA (Olds et al., 2002) and Finland (Aronen et al., 1996) have demonstrated long-term positive effects of extended postnatal home-visiting programmes. More recently, Dodge et al. (2014) showed the positive impact of postnatal home visiting on emergency medical care and in promoting more community connections, more positive parenting behaviours, and lower rates of anxiety among mothers (Dodge, 2014). In a review study of home-visiting programmes, Peacock et al. (2013) found a stronger positive effect of such programmes in certain disadvantaged populations.

Starting in 2013, and with financial support from the Public Health Agency of Sweden, an extended postnatal home-visiting programme was initiated in Rinkeby. The programme offers five extra home visits to all parents of a first child aged two to fifteen months, who attend Rinkeby Child Health Centre (Burström et al., 2017b). The overall purpose is to support and strengthen parents in their new role. The home visits are carried out by a child health nurse and a parental advisor from the social services. In the first phase of the programme, some 94% of such parents agreed to participate (Burström et al., 2017b).

The study design of the extended home-visiting programme in Rinkeby is not a randomized trial, but an intervention which is offered to all. A nearby clinic, as a control area for comparison, offers standard care. The content of the home visits is based on the national recommendations for child healthcare, but has been shaped by the participating child health nurses and parental advisors, who have developed and published a printed guideline of what to cover during the visits.

The visits have a natural progression, based on the child's age and developmental stage. Much of the content of the visits is guided by the parents' questions, and issues of attachment between mother (father) and child, child feeding, child safety, and so on can be informally discussed in the home environment. A recent qualitative evaluation of the content (Barboza et al., 2018) found that it covered all the domains of nurturing care as recommended both by the WHO Commission on Social Determinants of Health and by recent research (Britto et al., 2017). The content of the home visits can be understood as creating enabling conditions for health equity effects (Barboza et al., 2018).

In addition, other local community facilities such as the local library, dental services, and open childcare services are engaged in the project. Each child is given a picture book by the library, to promote early reading. The library also lends age-matched toys to families who cannot afford to buy the toys. The dental clinic provides a toothbrush to each child to promote dental hygiene. Open childcare services offer a stimulating daytime environment for both parents and their young children (Burström et al., 2017b).

The home-visiting programme has so far been successful. Participation rates are high, and parents are positive about the intervention and satisfied with the services offered. Participating staff like the way of working, and express that they are able to spend more time with parents with greater needs. Staff are also positive about the complementary skills provided by the child health nurse and the parental advisor in each team. The measles/mumps/rubella immunization rates have increased and there are indications of increased trust in healthcare services among parents, and some indication of lower rates of emergency ward visits. The home visits are a service offered to all, but are provided with greater intensity to those with greater needs (Burström et al., 2017b).

The extended home-visiting programme has caught the interest also of the national government, which decided in 2017 to allocate SEK 120 million (approximately 10 million pounds sterling) to expanding the programme to other areas of the country.

3.5 Looking forward to improved equity in healthcare

Healthcare systems in most high-income countries have traditionally been set up to deal with and treat acute illnesses. However, with improvements in the success of treatments and increased longevity, more people are living longer with chronic diseases and needing long-term contact with healthcare services. Increasingly, treatments and care may be provided in the home. A growing proportion of older people also have more than one disease, and may need attention from different medical specialists, as well as coordination between healthcare and social care services.

In a publicly funded healthcare system there may be trade-offs to be made between different objectives in delivering healthcare: for instance, between efficiency and equity, or between choice and fairness. What priority should be given to different objectives? What processes should be used to establish such priorities? In a publicly funded system, the public, as well as public health professionals working in the system, should obviously have an important role in deciding priorities. Another issue is who should provide the care, and how. Market mechanisms and privatization of the provision of care are not likely to achieve efficient and equitable care for those with the greatest need.

Recent reforms in health and social care in Sweden have focused on increasing patients' choice of providers, which may not be the highest priority for people with complex needs. It is important that policy makers realize that the major consumers of health and social care are older people with complex needs—and design services accordingly. Rather than emphasizing choice reforms as a solution for such older people, integration of different levels of healthcare services, as well as coordination between health and social care, may be more important for these individuals, and their spouses and relatives.

In addition, health policy makers should take into account that needs, and the use made of healthcare services, vary across population groups. Need is not always expressed in demand or use of care. Therefore different approaches, including outreach activities to people who need but, for different reasons, do not seek care, are required to meet the needs of different population groups. People living in disadvantaged areas and recent immigrants are examples of groups that require particular attention.

References

Adams, R.J., Stocks, N.P., Wilson, D.H., & Hill, C.L. (2009). Health literacy—a new concept for general practice? *Aust Fam Physician*, 38, 144–147.

Agerholm, J., Bruce, D., Ponce de Leon, A., & Burström, B. (2015). Equity impact of a choice reform and change in reimbursement system in primary care in Stockholm. *BMC Health Serv Res*, 15, 420.

Aronen, E.T. & Kurkela, S.A. (1996). Long-term effects of an early home-based intervention. *J Am Acad Child Adolesc Psychiatry*, 35, 1665–1672.

Barboza, M., Kulane, A., Burström, B., & Marttila, A. (2018). A better start for health equity? Qualitative content analysis of implementation of extended postnatal home visiting in a disadvantaged area in Sweden. *Int J Equity Health*, 17(1), 42. doi: 10.1186/s12939-018-0756-6

Barr, B., Bambra, C., & Whitehead, M. (2014). The impact of resource allocation policy on health inequalities in England 2001–11: longitudinal ecological study. *BMJ*, 348, g3231. doi: 10.1136/bmj.g3231

Beiki, O., Hall, P., Ekbom, A., & Moradi, T. (2012). Breast cancer incidence and case fatality among 4.7 million women in relation to social and ethnic background: a population-based cohort study. *Breast Cancer Res*, 14(1), R5.

Björkenstam, E., Ljung, R., Burström, B., Mittendorfer-Rutz, E., & Weitoft, G.R. (2012). Quality of medical care and excess mortality in psychiatric patients—a nationwide register based study in Sweden. *BMJ Open*, e000778.

Britto, P.R., et al. (2017). Nurturing care: promoting early childhood development. *Lancet*, 389, 91–102.

Burström, B. (2009). Market-oriented, demand-driven health care reforms and equity in health and health care utilization in Sweden. *Int J Health Serv*, 39(2), 271–285.

Burström, B., Burström, K., Nilsson, G., Tomson, G., Whitehead, M., & Winblad, U. (2017a). Equity aspects of the Primary Health Care Choice Reform in Sweden—a scoping review. *Int J Equity Health*, 16(1), 29.

Burström, B., Marttila, A., Kulane, A., Lindberg, L., & Burström, K. (2017b). Practising proportionate universalism—a study protocol of an extended postnatal home visiting programme in a disadvantaged area in Stockholm, Sweden. *BMC Health Serv Res*, 17(1), 91. doi: 10.1186/s12913-017-2038-1

Carr–Hill, R.A., Maynard, A., & Slack R. (1990). Morbidity variation and RAWP. *J Epidemiol Community Health*, 44, 271–273.

Dahlgren, G. (2018). *När sjukvården blev en marknad—effekter och alternativ* [*When Health Care Became a Market—Effects and Alternatives*]. Stockholm: Premiss Förlag.

Diderichsen, F., Varde, E., & Whitehead, M. (1997). Resource allocation to health authorities: the quest for an equitable formula in Britain and Sweden. *BMJ*, 315, 875.

Dodge, K.A., Goodman, W.B., Murphy, R.A., O'Donnell, K., Sato, J., & Guptill, S. (2014). Implementation and randomized controlled trial evaluation of universal postnatal nurse home visiting. *Am J Publ Health*, 104, S136–S143.

Fritzell, S., Schultz, A., Bokedal, C., & Burström, B. (2016). *Erfarenheter från hälsofrämjande befolkningsinriktat arbete i primärvården vid sex vårdcentraler i socialt och ekonomiskt utsatta områden i Stockholms län, 2013–2015* [*Experiences from Population-Oriented Health Promotion in Primary Care at Six Primary Care Clinics in Socially and Economically Disadvantaged Areas in Stockholm County*]. Stockholm: Stockholm County Council.

Gravelle, H., et al. (2003). Modelling supply and demand influences for deriving a needs-based capitation formula. *Health Econ*, 12, 985–1004.

Gulliford, M. (2003). Equity and access to care. In: M. Gulliford & M. Morgan (eds) *Access to Care*. London: Routledge, pp. 36–60.

Isaksson, D., Blomqvist, P., & Winblad, U. (2016). Free establishment of primary care providers: effects on geographical equity. *BMC Health Serv Res*, 16, 28.

Morgan, M. (2003). Patients' help-seeking and access to health care. In: M. Gulliford & M. Morgan (eds) *Access to Care*. London: Routledge, pp. 61–83.

National Health Service (NHS). (2018). NHS allocations. Available at: https://www.england.nhs.uk/allocations/#formulae

Olds, D.L., et al. (2002). Enduring effects of prenatal and infancy home visiting by nurses on children: follow-up of a randomized trial among children at age 12 years. *Arch Pediatr Adolesc Med*, 164, 412–418.

Peacock, S., Konrad, S., Watson, E., Nickel, D., & Muhajarine, N. (2013). Effectiveness of home visiting programs on child outcomes: a systematic review. *BMC Public Health*, 13, 17.

Peterson, P.N., et al. (2011). Health literacy and outcomes among patients with heart failure. *JAMA*, 305, 1695–1701.

Ratzan, S.C. & Parker, R.M. (2000). Introduction. In: C.R. Selden, M. Zorn, S.C. Ratzan, & R.M. Parker (eds) *National Library of Medicine Current Bibliographies in Medicine: Health Literacy*. NLM Pub. No. CBM 2000–1. Bethesda, MD: National Institutes of Health, US Department of Health and Human Services.

Regeringen [Government of Sweden]. (2016). *Effektiv vård* [*Effective/efficient care*]. Report on government investigation. SOU 2016:2. Stockholm: Statens Offentliga Utredningar. Available at: http://www.sou.gov.se/wp-content/uploads/2016/01/SOU-2016_2_Hela4.pdf

Riksrevisionen [National Audit Office]. (2014). *Primärvårdens styrning—efter behov eller efterfrågan?* [*Primary Health Care Governance—Based on Need or Demand?*]. RiR 2014:22. Stockholm: Riksrevisionen.

Svallfors, S. & Tyllström, A. (2018). Resilient privatisation: the puzzling case of for-profit welfare providers in Sweden. *Soc Econ Rev*, 16, 1–21.

Tao, W., Agerholm, J., & Burström, B. (2016). The impact of reimbursement systems on equity in access and quality of primary care: a systematic literature review. *BMC Health Serv Res*, 16(1), 542.

Tao, W., Bruce, D., & Burström, B. (2015). *Områdesskillnader i sjukdomsförekomst i Stockholms län* [*Area Differences in Disease Prevalence in Stockholm County*]. Rapport 2015:1. Stockholm: Centrum för epidemiologi och samhällsmedicin. Available at: http://folkhalsoguiden.se/amnesomraden/jamlik-halsa/rapporter/omradesskillnader-i-sjukdomsforekomst

4

Involving patients and publics in healthcare

Christopher McKevitt, Nina Fudge, and Clémence Pinel

4.1 Introduction

Increasingly, patients and members of the public are called upon to participate actively in the production and maintenance of their own health as informed, engaged, and responsible citizens and patients. At the same time, they are also being encouraged to engage in processes and practices aimed at enhancing the health of patient populations and the wider public. Patient and public involvement (also referred to as participation or engagement) encompasses a range of practices across diverse areas of health: shared decision making and self-management (Bodenheimer et al., 2002; Salzburg Global Seminar, 2011); policy decision making and planning; health service development (Best et al., 2012; Richards et al., 2013); research to understand and improve health and healthcare (Department of Health, 2006a); governance and quality assurance (Ocloo & Fulop, 2012; Oliver et al., 2002); and community development to improve population health and well-being. These practices are intrinsic to what Palmer et al. (2019) have termed a participatory zeitgeist, 'a distinct cultural and political movement' that signals a shift in concepts and practices related to individual and population health. This shift raises wider questions about knowledge and expertise, responsibility and accountability, citizenship and political organization. For health professionals, the desire or requirement to involve patients and/or members of the public in health processes may signify a non-traditional way of working that promises much in terms of innovation and efficacy but also presents challenges. Despite the recent exponential increase in involvement activities, policies, and infrastructures to support these, and burgeoning academic and grey literatures on the topic, involvement remains an emergent field that is characterized by debate about its purposes, methods, and evidence base.

This chapter provides an overview of the field of involvement of patients and members of the public in relation to healthcare, focusing on some of the key areas of debate. It outlines:

- Definitions and terminology
- Rationales

Christopher McKevitt, Nina Fudge, and Clémence Pinel, *Involving patients and publics in healthcare* In: *Healthcare Public Health*. Edited by: Martin Gulliford and Edmund Jessop, Oxford University Press (2020). © Oxford University Press.
DOI: 10.1093/oso/9780198837206.003.0004.

- Policies at supranational, national, and local level
- Methods of involvement
- Challenges

4.2 The lexicon of involvement

For simplicity, this chapter adopts the term 'involvement' to refer to policy and practices related to healthcare policy and services. The field as a whole is characterized by a diverse and changeable terminology across domains (such as policy, service development, or research), agencies (such as health systems and organizations providing healthcare), and nations. A wide variety of terms is used to denote actors (for example, patient, service user, consumer, public, community) and practices (for example, involvement, engagement, participation). Similarly, the field is characterized by a wide variety of terms denoting methods of involvement that may or may not be distinct, such as consultation, deliberation, focus group, participatory methods, co-production, co-design, and so on, deriving from different traditions and disciplines, as well as diverse epistemological and political positions.

There have been some attempts to standardize the vocabulary. In relation to patient and public involvement in research processes, the United Kingdom (UK) agency INVOLVE (2019) proposes the following definitions:

- Involvement—where members of the public are actively involved in research projects and in research organizations.
- Participation—where people take part in a research study.
- Engagement—where information and knowledge about research is provided and disseminated.

It is unlikely that such efforts to standardize terminology have had universal purchase, and the literature continues to call for greater specificity in the choice of terms used. Authors advocating or reporting efforts to involve patients and the public do not always explicitly articulate what they intend by their choice of a particular term, or use the same term in a single context. This means that communicating involvement can be hampered by terms that may not necessarily be synonymous and whose political or practical intents may or may not be shared by interlocutors.

4.3 Defining involvement

In this chapter, we refer to involvement as any practice that invites patients and/or other members of the public normally without a recognized qualification in a clinical, research, policy, or managerial field to take part in aspects of healthcare decision making, planning, development, or governance. We recognize that individuals who respond to such an invitation may in fact have such professional qualifications: doctors, academics, health service managers, and politicians are also patients and members of the public. In general, involvement tends to imply that those who are involved are 'ordinary' people invited to take part on the basis of their naivety in relation to policy making, planning, or service development. Martin (2008) has drawn attention to inherent tensions in the involvement agenda concerning representativeness of those who are involved and the constitutive basis of their contribution, a point we return to below. A fundamental principle of involvement is that it gives voice to citizens—'lay people'—who traditionally might not have contributed to shaping healthcare policies and practices.

In this chapter, we exclude patients' involvement in their own healthcare where this refers to concepts such as shared decision making, person-centred care, or patient activation. We acknowledge that there may be an implicit or explicit assumption that 'active' involvement in one's own healthcare (for example, through adopting healthy lifestyles, improving health literacy, sharing decision making processes in consultations, or self-managing long-term conditions) is connected to involvement in healthcare development at a wider policy or systems level. Work from the USA explicitly situates patient and family engagement in 'direct care' within a framework of engagement that also encompasses involvement in organizational design and governance and in policy making. This framework is underpinned by the idea that engagement at all levels of practices and processes directed towards the production of health can be viewed as an innovation that challenges 'an older paradigm of a paternalistic clinician and system' (Carman et al., 2013, p. 228), and has the potential to improve outcomes through better systems of care while reducing healthcare costs.

4.4 Rationales for involvement

The idea that patients, consumers, or the public should be actively involved in health at individual, system, and societal levels—in the clinic, in policy making, and in health research processes—is by now orthodox in many nations. As the social science literature indicates (Brown et al., 2004), there is a long history of patients organizing themselves into activist groups, for example to challenge medical definitions and ways of working, to highlight the stigma associated with specific conditions, and to call for increased research and intervention for conditions perceived to have been ignored. The women's health movement, mental health and disability rights groups, and HIV/AIDS activism are obvious examples. The involvement agenda represents a departure from this tradition which Brown and colleagues (2004) have called Embodied Health Movements. Involvement represents, in part at least, an institutional response to activists seeking to influence official agendas and ways of working; and it is constituted as an invitation from state institutions to citizens to collaborate in its work. For this reason, it is worth considering the diverse rationales that underpin this development. We argue it is important to understand these different accounts before undertaking an involvement strategy since they imply different kinds of activity, proposed outcomes, and indicators of success. In this section, we identify the main types of rationale proposed by advocates of involvement, as well as critical accounts of why involvement has been promoted.

4.4.1 Main types of rationale for involvement

The two main rationales underpinning the arguments promoting involvement tend to emphasize, on the one hand, its benefits in terms of enhancing quality and relevance, and, on the other hand, an ethical duty in democratic societies to promote participation in the institutional and social life of such societies.

The 'quality' argument is premised on the idea that patients' experiences, needs, and priorities can inform decision making and help to develop services that are more responsive to their needs. This has long been articulated in UK health policy documents, with the promise that involvement will lead to improved services and better outcomes for patients. Involvement is seen as a way for patients to contribute a unique element, in the form of their experiential knowledge of having a particular condition or using health services and thereby gaining a personal perspective on the quality of that service. Caron–Flinterman et al. (2005) argued that the experiential knowledge of patients is valued as it is seen to bring something new to the table—a form of knowledge which professionals do not have.

Much of the user involvement literature takes the basic premise that it is right to open up decision making in research and service development to the people that are directly affected by research outcomes and services. Involvement is portrayed as a means of giving people a 'voice'. Where health services are primarily funded by tax payers or other mandated contributions, it is argued that people who contribute financially are entitled to say how their contributions should be spent. European policy at the supranational level enshrines the rights of citizens' participation and empowerment as core values in all health-related work, with nation states encouraged to enhance citizens' abilities to participate (European Commission, 2007).

Promoting involvement in health has also been understood as a way of invigorating public engagement with democratic processes—an end in its own right. Participation in civil society has been not only encouraged at all levels but has, since 2008, also been made a legal requirement across Europe under the Lisbon Treaty. In order to increase participatory democracy in the European Union (EU), the treaty states that every citizen should be given the right to participate in the democratic life of the union, that decisions should be taken as openly and closely as possible to the citizen, and that institutions should maintain an open, transparent, and regular dialogue with representative associations and civil society.

This institutional enthusiasm for involvement also draws on a different tradition arising from a concern with social justice. In the UK and elsewhere, much of the involvement literature takes, as its starting point, the now classic and influential work of Sherry Arnstein (1969) and her ladder of citizen participation. Developed in the context of urban redevelopment in response to the growing civil rights movement, this model sees participation as a proxy for power, with the level of citizen power or control equated with different 'levels' of involvement or participation. The heuristic device of the ladder posits ever increasing degrees of control in influence and decision-making power. Thus, the rungs of this ladder start at 'Manipulation' and 'Therapy' (described as forms of non-participation), through to 'Informing', 'Consultation', and 'Placation' (seen as tokenistic participation, since citizens are assumed to lack the power to challenge the status quo), culminating in forms of participation where citizens have control over decision making.

Notions of empowering patients and citizens are commonplace in health policy documents, with the promotion of strategies to reduce recourse to healthcare through responsible lifestyles, wise choices in shared decision making, and self-management by those with self-limiting and long-term conditions. Policy documents sometimes suggest that the involvement of patients and the public in developing services will assist in this shift of power and empower patients (Department of Health, 2006b).

4.4.2 Critical readings of involvement

The rise in user involvement has been linked to global, societal changes since the 1970s, from when it has become acceptable to question scientific and expert authority (Cowden & Singh, 2007). This is particularly relevant in healthcare, in light of multiple health 'scandals' throughout history. The Tuskegee Syphilis Study (1932–72) researched, but did not treat, African–American men with syphilis, long after a definitive cure for syphilis had been discovered (Jones, 1981). In the 1980s and 1990s, NHS hospitals, the Bristol Royal Infirmary and Alder Hey Children's Hospital, were the sites of research scandals arising from the retention by doctors of organs of deceased children without the knowledge or permission of their parents. These acts were described as challenging the moral authority of the medical professionals and NHS organizations involved (Lawrence, 2002). In these contexts, involvement can be seen as more than a means to enhance quality, but also as enabling participatory governance, to reinstate trust in institutions responsible for the planning and provision of healthcare.

Involvement also resonates with wider questions regarding knowledge production itself. There has long been concern with a loss of faith in science and scientists such that efforts were needed to restore public trust in science (House of Lords Select Committee on Science and Technology, 2000), for example through strategies to democratize science. The work of Nowotny and colleagues (2001) proposes a shift in the production of new scientific knowledge from Mode 1 science (traditional scientific practice) to Mode 2 science (characterized as multidisciplinary, socially distributed, and directed towards practical application). Mode 2 science is also characterized as emphasizing the engagement of wider actors, outside qualified scientists.

In contrast, some authors have argued that involvement is a way for those in positions of authority to reinforce existing institutionally defined power relations and to legitimize decision making (Contandriopoulos, 2004; Komporozos-Athanasiou et al., 2018). Support for unpopular decisions can be achieved through consultation with service users, even though the consultation terms may be biased towards the opinions of those agencies that desired and organized a consultation, and while the consultation might not result in actions in line with the views given by participants. Harrison and Mort (1998) characterize public and user involvement as a 'technology of legitimation' to which particular professional groups accord no intrinsic representative legitimacy but which they use to advance their own ambitions over those of other groups.

4.5 The policy context

Policy makers of all types are promoting the idea that patients, the public, and communities should be invited to be involved. At the international level, the World Health Organization (WHO) promotes 'community engagement', tracing this concern back to the Alma Ata Declaration of 1978, when 'community participation was determined as a fundamental component of primary health care' (WHO, 2019). Subsequently, 'this notion was revitalized as "engagement and empowerment" and became a core strategy of the WHO Framework on integrated people-centred health services (IPCHS) adopted by Member States in 2016' (WHO, 2019). The argument is that 'communities need to be at the centre of drives to improve the quality of health services, access and equity, and achieving universal health coverage (UHC)' (WHO, 2020). Community engagement is seen as particularly important 'for global public health, as countries face complex health challenges that stretch and test the capacity and resilience of health systems and the populations they serve' (WHO, 2020). WHO Europe embeds engagement in its partnership approach to its policy framework for the twenty-first century, arguing that partnerships between institutions, communities, citizens, and private stakeholders can help foster new insights into the local determinants of health, secure support for action, while contributing to the development of communities (WHO, 2013).

In the EU, patient involvement in health policy and healthcare systems is a feature of a number of policy documents and reports emanating from the European Commission and European patient umbrella organizations. The EU White Paper, *Together for Health: A Strategic Approach for the EU 2008–2013* (European Commission, 2007), outlined the need for citizens' and patients' participation and empowerment to be regarded as core values in all health-related work at the EU level, and for nation states to do more to enhance an individual's ability to take part. The European Patients Forum has, among its goals: 'To advance meaningful patient involvement in the development and implementation of health-related policies, programmes and projects in the EU' and 'To contribute to improvements in health systems that enable equitable access to sustainable and high-quality healthcare' (European Patients Forum, 2019). Patient involvement in clinical research is advanced through the EU Patients Academy, an umbrella organization of patient groups active in public health and health advocacy across Europe.

A number of nations have developed policies to promote the involvement of patients and citizens in health services. For example, New Zealand's 2016 Health Strategy (Ministry of Health, 2016) was developed with input from public consultations and identified 'people powered' development as one of its five strategic themes. While fo-cusing on individual health through strengthened health literacy, and on individual choices, the themes also include partnership 'with people to design care that better meets their needs and wants' (Ministry of Health, 2016, p. 16). Ireland's Department of Health and Children developed, in 2008, a *National Strategy for Service User Involvement in the Irish Health Service 2008–2013*, arguing that involvement 'will re-sult in more appropriate services of a higher quality with increased service user com-pliance and satisfaction' (Department of Health and Children, 2008, p. 7). Sweden's public health policy emphasizes participation in society as salutogenic in its own right, with citizen participation in health services 'aimed at influencing the service provision function' and 'part of a "consumerist" movement in Scandinavian welfare states' (Fredriksson et al., 2018, p. 472).

NHS England is required by the Health and Social Care Act of 2012 and its 2016 Amendment (Her Majesty's Government, 2012) to involve patients not only in their own healthcare (through, for example, shared decision making in clinical consult-ations) but also in health service commissioning. Specifically, the Act prescribes that NHS England organizations must make arrangements to ensure that patients (or those who might use NHS services) are involved in the development and consideration of proposals for changes in the planning of health services and in decision making that might affect them. The Act is not prescriptive about how patients and the public should be involved, referring to involvement as 'whether by being consulted or provided with information or in other ways' (Her Majesty's Government, 2012). NHS England policy documents point to a myriad of other ways in which people can be 'involved', arguing that 'patient and public participation is important because it helps us to im-prove all aspects of health care, including patient safety, patient experience and health outcomes—giving people the power to live healthier lives' (NHS England, 2019). In relation to primary care in the UK, all general practices have, since 2015, been required to establish a Patient Participation Group, with a very broad remit that includes 'pro-viding the patient perspective, promoting self-care among patients and other health matters such as improving communication between the practice and its patients, influ-encing the development of services, liaising with other organisations both statutory and voluntary, contributing to the gathering of patient views including supporting and publicising patient surveys, and encouraging research' (Wilkie, 2016, p. 548).

In England and Wales, the National Institute for Health and Care Excellence (NICE) has identified quality standards for community engagement in health services that task professionals with demonstrating engagement with the public in priority set-ting, monitoring and evaluating health initiatives, identifying capacity to deliver ini-tiatives, and ensuring that community members are recruited to take on 'peer and lay roles' in initiatives.

Health policy organizations also are promoting community and public engage-ment. For example, in the UK, the King's Fund and the Health Foundation have both produced documents designed to support initiatives to strengthen community en-gagement in health, identifying a range of engagement strategies.

4.6 Methods of involvement

When it comes to putting involvement into practice, it would seem that there is no shortage of methods that might be used. For example, the online resource, Participation Compass, identifies 57 different methods (as well as estimating the potential costs associated with each). Deciding which method to use in which circumstance may be hampered by a lack of evidence about which method is most effective, as several authors have reported. A systematic review by Li et al. (2015) concluded by calling for further research to isolate the most impactful methods of involving publics. Dalton et al. (2016) concluded that further research is needed to identify the impact of different methods of engaging service users in health service configuration.

A number of factors can inform the choice of involvement method to be used. These include the purpose of involvement: is the aim to inform, to gain consensus, to demonstrate or enable democratic participation, to draw on the experiential knowledge of patients, carers, and family members in informing service development, or to 'empower' individuals or communities in health practices? Or is it indeed a combination of such aims? Another factor concerns the specific population to be involved: is the target population a specific constituency, such as those with a particular health condition, people from identifiable communities, people from disadvantaged groups, or the 'public' in general? Practical considerations such as available resources (including time, personnel, and finance) are also important. It may also be advantageous to engage with individual members of the target group to advise on appropriate methods.

Table 4.1 presents examples of methods that have been used, organized by the broad scope of the involvement exercise.

4.7 Involvement challenges

The implementation of patient and public involvement across all domains of health service development and delivery is characterized by a range of challenges. In this section, we present four key challenges that are discussed in the literature.

Table 4.1 Examples of the scope and methods of involvement

Scope	Examples of methods
Information	Media, public meetings, arts-based projects
Consultation	Public meetings, surveys, focus groups
Deliberation	Delphi method, priority setting partnerships
Development	Experience-based co-design, co-production, action research
Governance	Lay membership on governance groups and committees

The first relates to who is involved: which patients, which members of the public, which community members are invited to participate, and which of these accept the invitation? Is inviting people as individuals the same as inviting them through their membership of organizations such as patient advocacy groups or other civil society organizations? Do 'community leaders' speak on behalf of all their community, including women or young people? Are people who choose to join advisory groups or committees 'typical' of patients or the public?

Frequently such questions turn on notions of representativeness, with the assumption that involvement by individuals should enable the representation of an imagined larger public. The rationale for involvement seeking to incorporate lay experiential knowledge into decision making and planning relies less on ideas of democratic participation and more on the need to draw on diverse forms of knowledge, which are not necessarily available to professionals when they alone develop health services. This has been characterized as a 'tension' between 'public involvement premised on broad-based representation of an entire public (whether 'citizens', 'potential patients', 'local community' or 'users of a service') and one which draws on the knowledge of a select few within it' (Martin, 2008, p. 36). This tension may be persistent given the ambiguous and multiple meanings ascribed to involvement and the divergent tasks it is called upon to perform. This does underscore the need for clarity about purpose when embarking on involvement activities in specific arenas and with specific populations.

A common complaint made about involvement is that it can be tokenistic rather than meaningful (Gibson et al., 2012; Ocloo & Fulop, 2012). What makes involvement tokenistic or indeed meaningful has not been clearly articulated. Tokenistic involvement may refer to consultations that are perceived as redundant, or where it is suspected that decisions have already been made; feeling that one's views are not being listened to; or being involved but not able to influence decisions (Fudge et al., 2008). In an effort to foster meaningful involvement, a number of principles underpinning what makes for 'good' involvement practice have been reported (although these tend to be procedural, for example 'involve early', 'involve deeply'). Such efforts to codify involvement in practice may go some way to setting standards for processes but may not entirely overcome the perceived risk that involvement can be tokenistic. Rather, failure to involve in a 'meaningful' way has been attributed to the different types of knowledge associated with experts and lay people (Ward et al., 2010), and the privileging of expert over experiential knowledge (Morrison & Dearden, 2013). Involvement methods used have been criticized for their failure to adopt democratic models (Ocloo & Matthews, 2016), ensuring that traditional models of decision making are maintained (Gibson et al., 2012). These critics thus emphasize the need to consider questions of what kinds of power are at stake, and what capacity lay and professional stakeholders have to exercise power in determining the logic underpinning the involvement agenda itself, as well as the specific involvement practices adopted.

A further challenge to involvement lies in the question of impact and its evidence. Currently, there is a concern that involvement should be able to demonstrate impact (for example on service quality, efficiency, or patient outcomes), but two failings have been identified: first, that published accounts of involvement report processes of involvement but fail to report on impact; and second, that methods of assessing impact are inadequate (Dalton et al., 2016; Staniszewska et al., 2008). An early review of patient involvement in planning and developing health services (Crawford et al., 2002) identified specific changes that were attributed to patient involvement, such as improved sources of information and extending opening times. The authors concluded that there was insufficient evidence to demonstrate that involvement improved quality. Later reviews have reached similar conclusions (Conklin et al., 2015; Mockford et al., 2012). Studies have also identified the need to produce evidence of the economic costs and benefits of involvement (Mockford et al., 2012; Pizzo et al., 2015).

In contrast, some have argued that since involvement is a normative (democratic or ethical) good in its own right (Conklin et al., 2015; Crawford et al., 2002), efforts to assess impact should not ignore assessment of the quality of the efforts to involve. Others have argued that the concern with impact, a construct derived from the physical sciences, is oriented towards a linear model of cause and effect. This may be misleading where complex and unpredictable social actions are at work, so that using the notion of impact itself may discount the social value of involvement (Edelman & Barron, 2016; McKevitt et al., 2018).

One response to the perceived imperative to quantify the impact of involvement processes has been to develop and finesse approaches to measurement, with numerous tools already available. Dukhanin et al. (2018) recently reviewed 199 papers that reported on 23 different tools used to evaluate patient involvement in healthcare organization and systems decision making. They used inductive content analysis to develop a taxonomy of 116 process and outcome domains and subdomains, thereby mapping out a very wide range of quality indicators that have been considered in evaluation. They also suggest that there is much work to be done to inform decisions about which evaluation tools to use, since little is known about their robustness and not all tools will capture all indicators considered important.

4.8 Conclusion

Globally, health policy makers and providers are promoting the idea that patients and members of the public should be actively involved in decision making, research processes, and governance arrangements directed towards the provision of healthcare. This chapter has provided an overview of the concepts, rationales, and practices underpinning patient and public involvement in healthcare. It has also identified a number of challenges in the field that indicate its emergent status, while it suggests that much remains to be done to clarify terminology, agree purposes, identify most effective methods for specific involvement tasks, and build an evidence base of effectiveness. These questions require not just testing of solutions to technical problems but also consideration of more fundamental problematics of a social kind, such as the features of participatory democracy, the relative value attributed to different types of knowledge and expertise, and the nature of power differentials that shape involvement practices and outcomes.

A number of current developments in involvement strategies are addressing some of these questions. For example, the notion of co-production is gaining traction in health service development and delivery, promoting the idea that health service users and providers are engaged in partnership to produce health while articulating some of the tensions related to power dynamics inherent in any involvement activity (Batalden et al., 2016). The model of experience-based co-design, used to reimagine the delivery of healthcare services, introduces new actors—including design experts—into involvement practices, expanding the range of stakeholders with a role to play. It has been proposed that social values, derived though public engagement, could be incorporated into decision-making processes about healthcare resource allocation, in addition to health economic models.

Involvement remains a logistical challenge. Future research into involvement practices will need to demonstrate how the ethical argument for involvement can be aligned with the quality argument, so that the involvement imperative can be directed towards achieving desirable and equitable health outcomes.

References

Arnstein, S.R. (1969). A ladder of citizen participation. *J Am Instit Plan*, 35(4), 216–224.

Batalden, M., et al. (2016). Coproduction of healthcare service. *BMJ Qual Safe*, 25(7), 509–517.

Best, A., Greenhalgh, T., Lewis, S., Saul, J.E., Carroll, S., & Bitz, J. (2012). Large-system transformation in health care: a realist review. *Milbank Q*, 90(3), 421–456.

Bodenheimer, T., Lorig, K., Holman, H., & Grumbach, K. (2002). Patient self-management of chronic disease in primary care. *JAMA*, 288(19), 2469–2475.

Brown, P., Zavestoski, S., McCormick, S., Mayer, B., Morello-Frosch, R., & Gasior Altman, R. (2004). Embodied health movements: new approaches to social movements in health. *Sociol Health Ill*, 26(1), 50–80.

Carman, K., et al. (2013). Patient and family engagement: a framework for understanding the elements and developing interventions and policies. *Health Aff*, 32(2), 223–231.

Caron-Flinterman, J., Broerse, J., & Bunders, J. (2005). The experiential knowledge of patients: a new resource for biomedical research? *Soc Sci Med*, 60(11), 2575–2584.

Conklin, A., Morris, Z., & Nolte, E. (2015). What is the evidence base for public involvement in health-care policy? Results of a systematic scoping review. *Health Expect*, 18(2), 153–165.

Contandriopoulos, D. (2004). A sociological perspective on public participation in health care. *Soc Sci Med*, 58(2), 321–330.

Cowden, S. & Singh, G. (2007). The 'user': friend, foe or fetish? A critical exploration of user involvement in health and social care. *Crit Soc Policy*, 27(1), 5–23.

Crawford, M., et al. (2002). Systematic review of involving patients in the planning and development of health care. *BMJ*, 325(7375), 1263.

Dalton, J., Chambers, D., Harden, M., Street, A., Parker, G., & Eastwood, A. (2016). Service user engagement in health service reconfiguration: a rapid evidence synthesis. *J Health Serv Res Policy*, 21(3), 195–205.

Department of Health. (2006a). *Best Research for Best Health. A New National Health Research Strategy.* London: Department of Health. Available at: https://assets.publishing.service.gov.uk/government/uploads/system/uploads/attachment_data/file/568772/dh_4127152_v2.pdf [accessed 27 March 2019].

Department of Health. (2006b). *A Stronger Local Voice: A Framework for Creating a Stronger Local Voice in the Development of Health and Social Care Services.* London: Department of Health.

Department of Health and Children. (2008). *National Strategy for Service User Involvement in the Irish Health Service 2008–2013.* Dublin: Department of Health and Children. Available at: https://www.hse.ie/eng/services/publications/your-service,-your-say-consumer-affairs/strategy/service-user-involvement.pdf [accessed 27 March 2019].

Dukhanin, V., Topazian, R., & Decamp, M. (2018). Metrics and evaluation tools for patient engagement in healthcare organization- and system-level decision-making: a systematic review. *Int J Health Policy Manag*, 7(10), 889–903.

Edelman, N. & Barron, D. (2016). Evaluation of public involvement in research: time for a major re-think? *J Health Serv Res Policy*, 21(3), 209–211.

European Commission. (2007). *Together for Health: A Strategic Approach for the EU 2008–2013.* Brussels: European Commission. Available at: https://ec.europa.eu/health/ph_overview/Documents/strategy_wp_en.pdf [accessed 27 March 2019].

European Patients Forum. (2019). *A Strong Patients' Voice to Drive Better Health in Europe.* Available at: http://www.eu-patient.eu/About-EPF/whoweare/ [accessed 27 March 2019].

Fredriksson, M., Eriksson, M., & Tritter, J.Q. (2018). Involvement that makes an impact on healthcare: perceptions of the Swedish public. *Scand J Public Health*, 46(4), 471–477.

Fudge, N., Wolfe, C., & McKevitt, C. (2008). Assessing the promise of user involvement in health service development: ethnographic study. *BMJ*, 336(7639), 313–317.

Gibson, A., Britten, N., & Lynch, J. (2012). Theoretical directions for an emancipatory concept of patient and public involvement. *Health*, 16(5), 531–547.

Harrison, S. & Mort, M. (1998). Which champions, which people? Public and user involvement in health care as a technology of legitimation. *Soc Policy Admin*, 32(1), 60–70.

Her Majesty's Government. (2012). *Health and Social Care Act 2012.* Available at: http://www.legislation.gov.uk/ukpga/2012/7/pdfs/ukpga_20120007_en.pdf [accessed 27 March 2019].

House of Lords Select Committee on Science and Technology. (2000). *Science and Technology— Third Report.* Available at: http://www.publications.parliament.uk/pa/ld199900/ldselect/ldsctech/38/3801.htm [accessed 27 March 2019].

Involve. (2019). *What is public involvement in research?* Available at: https://www.invo.org.uk/find-out-more/what-is-public-involvement-in-research-2/ [accessed 27 March 2019].

Jones, J.H. (1981). *Bad Blood: The Tuskegee Syphilis Experiment.* New York: Free Press.

Komporozos–Athanasiou, A., Fudge, N., Adams, M., & McKevitt, C. (2018). Citizen participation as political ritual: towards a sociological theorizing of 'health citizenship'. *Sociology*, 52(4), 744–761.

Lawrence, C. (2002). Alder Hey. *J Epidemiol Comm Health*, 56(1), 4–5.

Li, K., Abelson, J., Giacomini, M., & Contandriopoulos, D. (2015). Conceptualizing the use of public involvement in health policy decision-making. *Soc Sci Med*, 138, 14–21.

Martin, G.P. (2008). 'Ordinary people only': knowledge, representativeness, and the publics of public participation in healthcare. *Sociol Health Ill*, 30(1), 35–54.

McKevitt, C., et al. (2018). Patient, carer and public involvement in major system change in acute stroke services: the construction of value. *Health Expect*, 21(3), 685–692.

Ministry of Health. (2016). *New Zealand Health Strategy: Future Directions.* Available at: https://www.health.govt.nz/system/files/documents/publications/new-zealand-health-strategy-futuredirection-2016-apr16.pdf [accessed 26 March 2019].

Mockford, C., Staniszewska, S., Griffiths, F., & Herron–Marx, S. (2012). The impact of patient and public involvement on UK NHS health care: a systematic review. *Int J Qual Health Care*, 24(1), 28–38.

Morrison, C. & Dearden, A. (2013). Beyond tokenistic participation: using representational artefacts to enable meaningful public participation in health service design. *Health Policy*, 112(3), 179–186.

NHS England. (2019). *Why get involved?* Available at: https://www.england.nhs.uk/participation/why/ [accessed 27 March 2019].

Nowotny, H., Scott, P., & Gibbons, M. (2001). *Re-Thinking Science: Knowledge and the Public in an Age of Uncertainty.* Cambridge, UK: Polity Press.

Ocloo, J. & Matthews, R. (2016). From tokenism to empowerment: progressing patient and public involvement in healthcare improvement. *BMJ Qual Safe*, 25(8), 626–632.

Ocloo, J.E. & Fulop, N.J. (2012). Developing a 'critical' approach to patient and public involvement in patient safety in the NHS: learning lessons from other parts of the public sector? *Health Expect*, 15(4), 424–432.

Oliver, S., Entwistle, V., & Hodnett, E. (2002). Roles for lay people in the implementation of health care research. In: A. Haines & A. Donald (eds) *Getting Research Findings into Practice.* London: BMJ Publishing, pp. 86–94.

Palmer, V.J., et al. (2019). The participatory zeitgeist: an explanatory theoretical model of change in an era of coproduction and codesign in healthcare improvement. *Med Humanit*, 45(3), 247–257.

Pizzo, E., Doyle, C., Matthews, R., & Barlow, J. (2015). Patient and public involvement: how much do we spend and what are the benefits? *Health Expect*, 18(6), 1918–1926.

Richards, T., Montori, V.M., Godlee, F., Lapsley, P., & Paul, D. (2013). Let the patient revolution begin. *BMJ*, 346, f2614.

Salzburg Global Seminar. (2011). Salzburg statement on shared decision making. *BMJ*, 342, d1745.

Staniszewska, S., Herron-Marx, S., & Mockford, C. (2008). Measuring the impact of patient and public involvement: the need for an evidence base. *Int J Qual Health Care*, 20(6), 373–374.

Ward, P., et al. (2010). Critical perspectives on 'consumer involvement' in health research: epistemological dissonance and the know-do gap. *J Sociol*, 46(1), 63–82.

Wilkie, P. (2016). Patient participation groups in general practice: building better partnerships. *Br J Gen Pract*, 66(652), 548–549.

World Health Organization. (2013). *Health 2020: A European Policy Framework and Strategy for the 21st Century.* Copenhagen: WHO. Available at: http://www.euro.who.int/__data/assets/pdf_file/0011/199532/Health2020-Long.pdf?ua=1 [accessed 27 March 2019].

World Health Organization. (2019). *WHO Framework on Integrated People-Centred Health Services.* Available at: https://www.who.int/servicedeliverysafety/areas/people-centred-care/en/ [accessed 27 March 2019].

World Health Organization. (2020). *Community engagement for quality, integrated, people-centred and resilient health services.* Available at: https://www.who.int/servicedeliverysafety/areas/qhc/community-engagement/en/ [accessed 4 March 2020].

5

Populations, values, and health

Ethical implications of population healthcare

A.M. Viens

5.1 Introduction

Healthcare and public health are traditionally distinguished on the basis of the differences in their aims, approaches, and contexts. Healthcare is typically understood as being focused at the individual level, taking place in hospitals and clinics, centred on biomedical risk factors, and being predominantly concerned with providing therapeutic interventions to treat already existing disease. Public health is typically understood as being focused at the population level, taking place in the community and society, centred on social and environmental risk factors, and being predominantly concerned with preventing or mitigating the need to access healthcare in the first place. In practice, of course, there are a number of connections and overlaps that can make drawing firm lines between healthcare and public health blurred or even artificial. When it comes to understanding their ethical foundations and how we should approach justifying their respective activities, however, the differences between healthcare and public health are quite important. The development over the last 20 or 30 years of public health ethics, as a distinct subfield of bioethics, has shown the importance of the critical analysis of questions raised by public health as deserving different approaches and perspectives than that of clinical medicine (Coggon & Viens, 2017).

As public health ethics has matured, as an academic field of specialization (Powers & Faden, 2008; Dawson & Verweij, 2009; Coggon, 2012; Barrett et al., 2016) and area of public health practice (Public Health Ontario, 2012; World Health Organization, 2017), we have started to see more attention being paid to some of the ethical implications of particular domains of public health practice and policy making. For instance, we can notice a move away from general public health ethics frameworks (Kass, 2001; Upshur, 2002; Childress et al., 2002; Grill & Dawson, 2017) towards more domain-specific public health ethical frameworks (Thompson, 2006; Tannahill, 2008; Carter, 2011). Nevertheless, population healthcare is one domain of public health that has received almost no attention within the public health ethics literature. This chapter seeks to remedy this situation by setting out and examining some of the philosophical and ethical presuppositions made by population healthcare, and its implications for how we should understand the jurisdiction, aims, and

A.M. Viens, *Populations, values, and health* In: *Healthcare Public Health*. Edited by: Martin Gulliford and Edmund Jessop, Oxford University Press (2020). © Oxford University Press. DOI: 10.1093/oso/9780198837206.003.0005.

evaluation of population healthcare. There are important questions that remain un-answered that population healthcare must seek to provide if it wants to be viewed as ethically robust and legitimate.

5. 2 The jurisdiction of population healthcare

Population healthcare, sometimes synonymously called healthcare public health, is conceived as one of four domains of public health practice (UK Faculty of Public Health, 2015; Nottinghamshire Healthcare NHS Foundation Trust, 2018):

(i) **Wider Determinants of Health**—affecting upstream causes of ill health (improving education, employment, sense of community, access to services, housing, reducing poverty, violence, stigma, poor lifestyle opportunities);

(ii) **Health Improvement**—helping people make healthy behavioural choices—for patients and for staff;

(iii) **Health protection**—keeping people safe from infection, poor environment and injury;

(iv) **Healthcare Public Health/Population Healthcare**—making our services op-timal (effective and efficient) and accessible to all and benefitting the most number of people in need with the resources we have.

It is useful to understand the nature of population healthcare through the notion of jur-isdiction; the metaphor of jurisdiction can be helpful in elucidating where population healthcare operates, what authority it has, and the scope of its values. While the wider determinants of health are often beyond the direct jurisdiction of public health prac-titioners, population healthcare certainly provides an area whereby traditional health authorities have more influence. The jurisdiction of population healthcare is planted firmly within the healthcare system, while extending beyond the walls of clinics and hospitals, given the organized community and political efforts needed to maintain the healthcare system. The need for social coordination to bring about population health-care, especially the role of the government, speaks to the shared responsibility to assure the conditions under which people can be healthy and enjoy health equity.

The intersection of health services and public health is not novel to popula-tion healthcare, as evidenced by efforts to integrate primary care and public health (Institute of Medicine, 2012; Valaitis, 2012; Millar et al., 2014). Nevertheless, popula-tion healthcare seems to be more than just the integration of primary care and public health. According to Sir Muir Gray, 'Population healthcare and personalised care are two sides of the same coin. It's sometimes a different language, but it's the same cur-rency' (Gray, 2014). It is not exactly clear how this should shape our understanding of the jurisdiction of population healthcare. One way in which it appears it will have an important implication, however, will be in how we should be thinking about health and healthcare at the population level. Stein and Galea (2019) put the point well in elucidating the distinction between health and healthcare:

> Health is a desired state of wellbeing that allows us to do what we want to do, that has us living full, rich lives, achieving whatever potential we wish to achieve. Healthcare is the system that aims to restore us to health when we get sick ... The conflation of health and healthcare has resulted in a one-sided, indefatigable investment in healthcare. Yet this focus on curative medicine is not improving our health. We should be focusing on health, on keeping us healthy to begin with.

As such, without a clear understanding of the proper jurisdiction of population healthcare, we may risk creating a number of issues. First, we risk equating investment in healthcare with investment in health. As David Hunter maintains, 'There is a growing recognition in many countries that simply pouring resources into health care services, especially those centred on acute hospital care, cannot be equated with good health' (Hunter, 2008, p. 217). Second, and relatedly, we risk encouraging the problem of overstating healthcare as a determinant of health. While healthcare is important, as an area of public health practice itself, we must take seriously the extent to which we primarily focus on it as a determinant of health for the entire population. Third, public health institutions and activities have been notoriously underfunded, so if investment in population healthcare counts as investment in public health, then it risks drawing much needed resources away from traditional areas of public health practice.

In order to have a better sense of how population healthcare might face such issues, we will need to examine its aims more closely. As I have argued elsewhere, 'the social mission and social machinery needed to understand and advance the state's health responsibilities to assure conditions under which people can be healthy establishes a key role for political morality in determining what forms and means of co-ordination is required to meet these responsibilities' (Viens, 2019, p. 147). Through a better understanding of the values of population healthcare and the value it seeks to promote, we will be able to achieve a clearer picture of some of the ethical questions it raises.

5.3 The aim of population healthcare

According to the UK Faculty of Public Health (2017, p. 1), population healthcare is:

> concerned with maximising the population benefits of healthcare and reducing health inequalities while meeting the needs of individuals and groups, by prioritizing available resources, by preventing diseases and by improving health-related outcomes through design, access, utilisation and evaluation of effective and efficient health and social care interventions, settings and pathways of care.

According to Public Health England (Gray, 2014), the aim of population healthcare is:

> to maximise value and equity by focusing not on institutions, specialties or technologies, but on populations defined by a common symptom, condition or characteristic, such as breathlessness, arthritis, or multiple morbidity.

Within these definitions, we see a clear articulation of both the main aims of population healthcare and the means by which it seeks to accomplish these aims. The dual aims of maximizing population benefits of healthcare and reducing health inequalities are clearly moral aims—namely, well-being (of which health is a key constituent) and justice (of which equity is a key concern). The means—through prioritizing resources (justice), preventing disease (well-being), and improving design, access, utilization, and evaluation (efficiency)—are also moral considerations. Each of the values which seek to guide and define the mission of population healthcare, and the means by which population healthcare will achieve its mission, carry ethical implications worthy of further examination.

The value of promoting health and well-being is traditionally understood as a consequentialist moral concern. On this view, we ought to be guided by practices and policies that promote good consequences, such as good health outcomes. We see the predominance of consequentialist thinking in the utilitarian basis of health economic evaluation and resource allocation predicated on cost–benefit analysis. While the focus on maximizing overall benefit for the entire population has tended to give public health practice a largely consequentialist appearance, public health is also guided by other values. The value of protecting health equity is traditionally understood as a deontological moral concern. According to this, we ought to be guided by practices and policies that promote our duties and respect the rights of others. We see the importance of deontological thinking in efforts to reduce health inequalities and in a greater focus on securing the human right to health. It is clear that, as these two central ethical values of public health have their basis in two different ethical theories, there is a risk of conflicting ideas and goals—and, in such circumstances, a need to find a way to balance and make trade-offs between these different ethical values.

Nevertheless, we see within the development of population healthcare how these underlying principles drive the types of value it seeks to promote. Under the conception of population healthcare advanced by Gray and his colleagues (Gray, 2011; Gray et al., 2017), there are three dimensions of value that population healthcare seeks to advance:

(i)   **Allocative value**—the value obtained from how well resources are *distributed* to different subgroups within the population.
(ii) **Technical value**—the value obtained from how well resources are satisfying the *needs* of the population.
(iii) **Personalized value**—the value obtained from how well the outcomes relate to the values of each individual within the population.

It should be clear that when 'value' is used in this context, it references to outcomes in relation to cost (Porter, 2010; Volpp et al., 2012). Thus, while population healthcare as a domain of public health is guided by the two central ethical values of promoting health and health equity, these values are constrained by how well resources are distributed to the satisfaction of patient needs and preferences. This is going to have an impact on how we understand and evaluate the ethics of population healthcare. Of particular concern is how we understand personalized value and its role in justifying population healthcare interventions.

Bringing about personalized value will be accomplished through satisfying individual patients; in particular, the value that is obtained from how well the improvement in health outcomes relates to the personal values and preferences of each individual within the population. This would make it distinct, as an ethical concern, from the primary values of promoting health and health equity, yet these are related insofar as they are connected to the individual judgement of patients in relation to their experienced health outcomes. This, of course, raises a number of ethical and philosophical questions. While it is true that patients are more likely to comply with treatment recommendations that are based on their values and preferences, to what extent should individual patient preferences be taken into account for population-level decisions? What if individuals do not have an interest in being healthy or seeing an equitable distribution of health status or outcomes across the population? To what extent should such preferences be taken into account with those who share opposing views? How should we adjudicate differences and conflicts between the primary values of well-being and justice, and personal preferences? Is it not an unfair instance of double counting for both technical and personalized value, which both focus on patient outcomes (i.e. the satisfaction of needs versus the satisfaction of preferences), against the weight of allocative value?

There are also important questions to be raised about the extent to which we should think these allocative, technical, and personalized values are in anyway comparable or commensurate (Elster & Roemer, 1993; Hausman, 1995; Chang, 1998). This is going to be a key consideration within population healthcare policy and its task of weighing and balancing these values against each other in making commissioning decisions. One thing that seems evident in population healthcare is that (a) it does not treat health as a value *in itself*, let alone a value to be maximized independent of healthcare, and (b) it does not provide us with an independent means for valuing an equitable distribution. We seem to only value distribution insofar as it helps us improve overall health outcomes. Making health outcomes the primary currency through which a value-based, population healthcare approach is maintained runs the risk of making it more difficult to justify than the best use of finite resources. There is not a simple direct correlation between improving healthcare delivery and better health outcomes. The distribution of benefits, and how we should balance the benefits and burdens needed to achieve such outcomes, is a complex question that requires a better understanding of how the different dimensions of value that are at the core of population healthcare should operate.

As we have seen, population healthcare is committed to both promoting technical value (health) and allocative value (health equity), but how should it deal with situations when these values are in tension or cannot be mutually achieved to the same extent? What is a fair way of reaching resource allocation decisions? For example, what priority should be given to reducing inequalities over increasing overall health gains? Or to the benefits for a small number of very high-cost patients, as compared to smaller benefits for the many? Or to the growing numbers of very elderly people requiring care towards the end of their lives? These are all questions that can only be answered by public health ethics. It is evident that much of the development of population healthcare has proceeded with little engagement with the public health ethics literature, which has sought to answer these very questions.

We might also worry how population healthcare will face traditional ethical issues about autonomy versus paternalism, especially in light of population healthcare's focus on personalized value and patient preference. Within the healthcare setting, autonomy tends to take precedence and hence becomes a primary focus of medical ethics. It has become a dominant value within bioethics more generally, which creates important problems for how we conceive of public health ethics (Dawson, 2010). This creates a serious challenge for population-level health interventions that we know will improve the public's health but can be controversial or even harmful for some individuals. How should, for instance, population healthcare ethically address preventive medicine and screening? On what basis should it seek to balance the technical value that can be obtained from population screening versus over-diagnosis and other harms, or ensure the allocative value of screening which often benefits the least advantaged to a much lesser degree? (Newson, 2011) The use of antenatal and genetic screening raises a number of ethical issues that population healthcare will need to address, and with its central focus on the ethical values of protecting health and promoting health equity, yet also seeking to include patient preferences, it is going to require a clear accounting of how much deference should be provided to autonomy and personalized value in light of what can be gained in both technical and allocative value with population screening.

5.4 The evaluation of population healthcare

It is maintained that a value-based approach to healthcare, of which population healthcare is an instance, is 'the equitable, sustainable and transparent use of the available resources to achieve better outcomes and experiences for every person' (Hurst, 2019). This is not only an immense promise, it is one that is fundamentally moral—equity, sustainability, transparency, and betterness are all normative concepts. In order to evaluate the extent to which population healthcare can deliver on such a promise, we are going to need an idea of how we should measure and demonstrate how its activities are improving health outcomes, reducing health inequalities, and aligning with individual preferences.

As noted earlier in Section 5.3, Gray et al. (2017) identify three different types of value that population healthcare should be concerned with when seeking to measure and demonstrate its effectiveness:

(i)   **Allocative value**—which is measured in terms of *equity*.
(ii) **Technical value**—which is measured in terms of *outcomes*.
(iii) **Personalized value**—with no mention of how this is to be measured.

Our ability to promote allocative value from population healthcare interventions will depend on how well resources are distributed in terms of mitigating differences in health between and among population groups. That will depend on what makes the inequity in health outcomes unjust and meriting response. In order to evaluate how well we are doing in promoting allocative value, we need to know what we should be aiming at. Should we be aiming at equality, in which every member of the relevant population has the same outcomes? Should we be aiming at sufficiency, in which, while not every member has the same outcomes, they all achieve a basic level of health outcomes? Should we be aiming at the least advantaged, in which we ensure that those who are worst off are given the greatest priority when distributing resources within the population? Population healthcare cannot make such assessments itself; it must seek the help of moral and political philosophy to provide the criteria that should be used to make these normative judgements.

Our ability to promote technical value from population healthcare interventions will depend on how we define the needs of the population. On the one hand, we will want to know whether needs are confined to traditional healthcare resources, such as access to primary care services, or whether needs will also include access to resources and opportunities that are conducive to bringing about health, such as stable income, housing, and vocational/educational opportunities. On the other hand, we will also want to know whether we are understanding needs as being objective or subjective in nature. If needs are objective, then there are certain considerations required by all humans, by virtue of their nature, that we may seek to promote throughout the population. If needs are subjective, however, then what is needed by individuals within a population will be relative and will depend on individual preferences. This is going to matter because, while the definition of technical value refers to resources, it is to be evaluated in terms of outcomes. If our ability to promote technical value will be evaluated in terms of health status outcomes, then this is going to influence what measures we should adopt. For instance, imagine that we seek to evaluate the satisfaction of needs in terms of measuring the quality of life of patients. If we take a subjective approach, seeking to evaluate patient preference satisfaction as evidence of their overall quality of life—such as quality adjusted life years (QALYs) assessments—then this is going to have a big impact on how we seek to maximize technical value.

Our ability to promote personalized value will be more difficult. Unlike allocative and technical value, which proponents of population healthcare have been clear on how they should be measured, personalized value does not have an obvious metric.

In order to know how well the outcomes relate to the values and preferences of each individual within the population, we need to know whether it is only for the individual to know/decide when outcomes align with their values—as well as whether there are means of determining the preference satisfaction of each individual within a population without having to ask each individual (which would be a massive time and resource expense). Moreover, there are two large challenges that will confront our ability to use personalized value within population healthcare. First, people are often poor arbiters of their preferences. The notion of personalized value presupposes that preferences are clear, stable, and true reflections of what individuals value. Second, people often shape their preferences to their socioeconomic circumstance, which risks perpetuating further inequalities between members of the population. As we know from Amartya Sen's work on adaptive preferences, there can be objectively unhealthy individuals who believe their health is fine and are satisfied with their health status despite suffering material deprivation and social injustice (Sen, 1992, 1999).

5.5 Conclusion

According to Gray (2014), 'population healthcare offers us the opportunity to increase the value of available resources in a way that will not be possible through a more intense focus on the bureaucracies that have served us well, but which are insufficient to meet the challenges of the 21st century'. While population healthcare seeks to ensure that our healthcare services are effective and efficient, it also must ensure such services are ethical. In order to do so, they need to provide, inter alia, equitable access to all in a way that can seek to benefit the greatest number of people, especially the least advantaged. If population healthcare is to be one of the domains of public health practice—which was notably characterized by Winslow (1920) as comprising both an art and science—it will have its work cut out for it. The significant improvements in value promised by population healthcare will require a fundamental reinvestment and restructuring of healthcare delivery, including finding a way to strike the difficult balance between addressing the social determinants of health that have the greatest impact on a population's health and patient perspectives that healthcare is the most important determinant of health.

This is a challenging mission—especially in light of the serious resource and personnel constraints facing the health service, only magnified further under conditions of austerity in places like the UK. What is essential to recognize is that the mission of population healthcare, as we have observed by examining its jurisdiction and aims, is fundamentally ethical. In order to succeed in its mission, practitioners and policy makers that work and administer the various components of population healthcare need to understand how the ethical values of promoting health and health equity (along with others) contribute to both justifying and guiding its activities.

There also remain some wider questions within public health ethics regarding how we should understand population healthcare, and its interconnections with the other domains of public health practice. In particular, it would be beneficial to see more work developing on what relative weight we should accord to allocative, technical, and personalized value, and the relative priority that should be assigned to population healthcare compared to other domains of public health practice. Given the importance of prevention and the wider determinants of health, and the recent disinvestment in traditional public health domains, it remains a key ethical and policy question just how much of our efforts and resources should be focused on healthcare compared to health at the population level.

References

Barrett, D.H., Ortmann, L.H., Dawson, A., Saenz, C., Reis, A., & Bolan, G. (eds) (2016). *Public Health Ethics: Cases Spanning the Globe*. Cham, CH: Springer.

Carter, S.M., et al. (2011). Evidence, ethics, and values: a framework for health promotion. *Am J Public Health*, 101, 465–472.

Chang, R. (1998). (ed.) *Incommensurability, Incomparability, and Practical Reason*. Cambridge, MA: Harvard University Press.

Childress, J., et al. (2002). Public health ethics: mapping the terrain. *J Law Med Ethics*, 30, 170–178.

Coggon, J. (2012). *What Makes Health Public? A Critical Evaluation of Moral, Legal, and Political Claims in Public Health*. Cambridge: Cambridge University Press.

Coggon, J. & Viens, A.M. (2017). *Public Health Ethics in Practice*. London: Public Health England.

Dawson, A. (2010). The future of bioethics: three dogmas and a cup of hemlock. *Bioethics*, 24, 218–225.

Dawson, A. & Verweij, M. (eds) (2009). *Ethics, Prevention, and Public Health*. Oxford: Oxford University Press.

Elster, J. & Roemer, J.E. (eds) (1993). *Interpersonal Comparisons of Well-Being*. Cambridge: Cambridge University Press.

Gray, M. (2014). Population based and personalised care—two sides of the same coin. *BMJ Opinion*, 4 July 2014. Available at: https://blogs.bmj.com/bmj/2014/07/04/muir-gray-population-based-and-personalised-care-two-sides-of-the-same-coin/

[As quoted in] Gray, M. (2014). Population health—what's in a name. *BMJ Opinion*, 4 June 2014. Available at: https://blogs.bmj.com/bmj/2014/06/04/muir-gray-population-health-whats-in-a-name/

Gray, J.A.M. (2011). *How to Get Better Value Healthcare* (2nd edn). Oxford: Offox Press.

Gray, J.A.M., Chana, N., & Kanani, N. (2017). Leadership of population healthcare. *J Roy Soc Med*, 110, 400–403.

Grill, K. & Dawson, A. (2017). Ethical frameworks in public health decision-making: defending a value-based and pluralist approach. *Health Care Anal*, 25, 291–307.

Hausman, D.M. (1995). The impossibility of interpersonal utility comparisons. *Mind*, 104, 473–490.

Hunter, D.J. (2008). Health needs more than health care: the need for a new paradigm. *Eur J Public Health*, 18, 217–219.

Hurst, L., et al. (2019). *Defining Value-Based Healthcare in the NHS*. Oxford: Centre for Evidence-Based Medicine. Available at: https://www.cebm.net/wp-content/uploads/2019/04/Defining-Value-based-healthcare-in-the-NHS_201904.pdf

Institute of Medicine. (2012). *Primary Care and Public Health: Exploring Integration to Improve Population Health*. Washington, DC: The National Academies Press.

Kass, N. (2001). An ethics framework for public health. *Am J Public Health*, 91, 1776–1782.

Millar, J., Bruce, T., Cheng, S.M., Masse, R., & McKeown, D. (2014). Is public health ready to participate in the transformation of the healthcare system? *Healthc Pap*, 13, 10–21.

Newson, A.J. (2011), Population screening. In A. Dawson (ed.) *Public Health Ethics: Key Concepts and Issues in Policy in Practice*. Cambridge: Cambridge University Press, pp. 118–142.

Nottinghamshire Healthcare NHS Foundation Trust. (2018). *Strategic Public Health Framework Update: Improving the Health of the Public and Reducing Inequality Through the Work of the Trust*. Nottingham: Nottinghamshire Healthcare NHS Foundation Trust.

Porter, M.E. (2010). What is the value in health care? *New Engl J Med*, 363, 2477–2481

Powers, M. & Faden, R. (2008). *Social Justice: The Moral Foundations of Public Health and Health Policy*. Oxford: Oxford University Press.

Public Health Ontario. (2012). *A Framework for the Ethical Conduct of Public Health Initiatives*. Toronto: Public Health Ontario.

Sen, A. (1992). *Inequality Reexamined*. Cambridge, MA: Harvard University Press.

Sen, A. (1999). *Commodities and Capabilities*. Oxford: Oxford University Press.

Stein, M. & Galea, S. (2019). A party trick. *Public Health Post*, 4 April 2019. Available at: https://www.publichealthpost.org/the-publics-health/a-party-trick/

Tannahill, A. (2008). Beyond evidence–to ethics: a decision-making framework for health promotion, public health and health improvement. *Health Prom Int*, 23, 380–390.

Thompson, A.K., Faith, K., Gibson, J.L., & Upshur, R.E.G. (2006). Pandemic influenza preparedness: an ethical framework to guide decision-making. *BMC Med Ethics*, 7, 12.

UK Faculty of Public Health. (2015). *Short Headline Definition of Healthcare Public Health*. London: Faculty of Public Health.

UK Faculty of Public Health. (2017). *Health Services Committee. Healthcare Public Health*. London: Faculty of Public Health. Available at: https://www.fph.org.uk/media/1879/hcph-definition-final.pdf

Upshur, R. (2002). Principles for the justification of public health intervention. *Can J Public Health*, 93, 101–103.

Valaitis, R. (2012). *Strengthening Primary Health Care through Primary Care and Public Health Collaboration*. Ottawa, ON: Canadian Health Services Research Foundation.

Viens, A.M. (2019). Neoliberalism, austerity and the political determinants of health. *Health Care Anal*, 27(3), 147–152.

Volpp, K.G., Loewenstein, G., & Asch, D.A. (2012). Assessing value in health care programs. *JAMA*, 307, 897–899.

Winslow, C.-E.A. (1920). The untilled fields of public health. *Science*, 51(1306), 23–33.

World Health Organization. (2017). *WHO Guidelines on Ethical Issues in Public Health Surveillance*. Geneva: WHO.

6
Healthcare needs assessment

Andrew O'Shaughnessy and John Wright

6.1 Introduction

Meeting the healthcare needs of individuals and populations is a key aim of delivering population-based healthcare. Healthcare needs assessment (HCNA) is a method for developing public health advice and incorporating this into the planning and commissioning of health services. HCNA draws on the thinking of a wide range of actors: philosophers and economists have discussed the definition and meaning of the word 'need' and how this should be measured; health providers have interests in supplying services for the diagnosis and treatment of particular diseases; patients and the public have specific wants and demands that they consider should receive priority. Measuring the health needs of individuals and communities can address these different viewpoints by providing evidence to inform the planning and provision of health services and ensuring the efficient and equitable use of health resources (Wright et al., 1998). In health systems with population-based primary care, the gatekeeping role of primary care physicians regulates access to specialist and hospital-based care. Here, needs assessment for individuals and practice populations is of daily relevance but may not always be operationalized explicitly, leading to wide variations in practice (Wilkinson & Murray, 1998).

6.2 Rationale for needs assessment

HCNA was first advocated in the UK, in the 1989 White Paper *Working for Patients* (Department of Health, 1989), which introduced the separation of purchaser and provider functions as a central element of a new strategy to increase efficiency or 'value for money' in the health service. The purchaser function became the new responsibility of health authorities and their successors (presently, clinical commissioning groups), while the provider function was to be discharged by hospitals and community services. On the purchaser side, systematic use of HCNA was intended to guarantee that contracts could be set in place to ensure that healthcare services met the health needs of local populations. This contrasted with the pre-existing arrangement in which health authorities were given funds to run hospital services, perpetuating historical inequalities in the supply of services and sometimes promoting supplier-induced demand. On the provider side, the White Paper controversially promoted market-style competition between providers through an internal market in services.

Andrew O'Shaughnessy and John Wright, *Healthcare needs assessment* In: *Healthcare Public Health*. Edited by: Martin Gulliford and Edmund Jessop, Oxford University Press (2020). © Oxford University Press. DOI: 10.1093/oso/9780198837206.003.0006.

The reforms also aimed to promote patient choice and improved service quality, with funding following patients to their preferred provider. While the internal market has not endured in the UK, the concept of population-based HCNA to inform health service commissioning and planning has continuing relevance in any jurisdiction.

6.3 Development of needs assessment

In order to support the healthcare reforms, the Department of Health in England established a programme of applied research and development to contribute to an evidence-based approach to healthcare. As part of this programme, Stevens et al. (2004) developed methods for HCNA and worked with a wider group of authors to produce a series of needs assessments across different areas of healthcare. The publication of these assessments, in a three-volume book, ushered in a new phase in the development and legitimacy of needs assessment methods (Stevens et al., 2004). A series of papers was published in the BMJ (Wright et al., 1998). These publications focused on equipping the new commissioners and their public health advisers with the tools to accurately and fairly direct health resources towards those population groups where healthcare needs are greatest. HCNA should explicitly identify measures required to promote equity and reduce inequalities, as well as increasing effectiveness and efficiency. This chapter draws on these earlier texts, which remain relevant today, even though some elements of the commissioning and policy landscape have changed.

6.4 The contemporary context

National, regional, and local studies to help maximize the efficiency and fairness of health and social care services are now of great relevance. The rapid increase in life expectancy in recent decades has resulted in people over 80 years old now representing the fastest growing sector of the population (Hazra & Gulliford, 2017). This has been accompanied by an apparent expansion of morbidity. People live longer with multiple long-term conditions that can be treated, but not cured, through healthcare intervention. The prevalence of multimorbidity increases substantially with age and is present in most people aged 65 years and over. There is good evidence that the number of conditions can be a greater determinant of a patient's use of health service resources than the specific diseases involved themselves (Barnett et al., 2012).

Increasing consumerism, and the more democratic expression of opinion through social media, have enabled members of the public to give expression to their expectations and concerns about the quality of the services they receive, from access and equity, to appropriateness and effectiveness. Health and social care systems continue to adopt new innovations and costly technological advances against an uncertain economic and political background and significant workforce pressures. Precise, pragmatic, and practical solutions or, as a minimum, mitigations, are essential to help ensure that health and social care services continue to meet the needs of the population. Despite efforts to rebalance resource allocation, the 'inverse care law' is still apparent (Tudor Hart, 2000), and there is wide variation in availability and use of healthcare by geographical area and point of provision (Wright et al., 1998).

6.5 Definition of need

Need in healthcare is commonly defined as the **capacity to benefit** from healthcare intervention (Stevens et al., 2004). This requires two conditions: the existence of a health problem and the potential for effective intervention to improve health status. Ill health alone cannot be equated with need because the identification of 'need' also requires the potential to improve health through intervention. From a health economic perspective, the concept of need as capacity to benefit must also be qualified by the resources required to improve health. If a person might gain the same health benefit either from a less costly intervention or a more costly intervention, the latter cannot be justified ethically and is not needed (Culyer & Wagstaff, 1993). A similar consideration applies in addressing the needs of two different individuals. One individual might need a cost-effective treatment but, if there are diminishing marginal returns as treatment progresses, the incremental cost of restoring the individual to complete health might not be justified when compared with initiating treatment for another person with different needs. Culyer (1998) suggested that need is not simply the capacity to benefit but should be defined as 'the amount and type of health care that is necessary to eliminate a person's capacity to benefit from it in terms of health gain', with only cost-effective care being considered relevant in the context of this definition.

Epidemiologists and health economists have different approaches to defining health priorities. An epidemiologist may consider that measures of the burden of disease—such as incidence, prevalence, mortality, and disability adjusted life years (DALYs)—are indicators of need, with the leading causes of death or DALYs being ranked as the highest priorities. From a health economic perspective, needs should be ranked in terms of the incremental costs and benefits from intervention, with the intervention strategies with the lowest cost per quality adjusted life year (QALY) receiving the highest priority (Donaldson & Mooney, 1991). In drawing on these approaches, public health is adopting the utilitarian ethical objective of maximizing the health gain that can be obtained from available resources across entire populations. But, as we note in other chapters in this volume, reducing inequalities and promoting equity are also important and sometimes competing goals.

6.6 Different aspects of needs

Assessing needs according to the theoretical definitions previously outlined requires a sophisticated level of subject-specific knowledge that may not always be available.

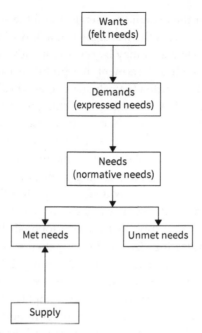

Figure 6.1 Different aspects of need.

Adapted with permission from Wright et al. 'Development and importance of health needs assessment.' *BMJ*, Vol. 316, Issue 7140, pp. 1310–13. Copyright © 1998 BMJ Publishing Group Ltd.

Bradshaw (1972) suggested four types of need that can be applied in practice (Figure 6.1). Needs defined by experts are referred to as 'normative needs' (Bradshaw, 1972). Normative needs are not measured in absolute terms because standards for assessment may vary depending on the experts consulted. 'Comparative needs' depend on comparing the care received by different but equivalent groups of patients. Individuals and communities may have 'felt needs', which depend on the perceptions of individuals or communities of their needs. These may be turned into 'expressed needs' if perceptions of need are translated into help-seeking behaviours. However, people may have health needs that they are unaware of, and for which they might benefit from healthcare intervention. Such unfelt and unexpressed needs can sometimes be identified through opportunistic testing in primary care or through national screening programmes. A person who has their blood pressure measured may be surprised to find that they have hypertension, a largely asymptomatic condition.

6.7 Need, demand, and supply

Needs assessment is sometimes used to inform the design of a completely new service, but it is more common to use it to evaluate what incremental changes can be made to existing services. Here, it is important to consider how the need for healthcare overlaps with the demand for services and the supply of healthcare. In economics, 'demand' represents the willingness or ability of individuals or families to consume healthcare. Demands may be consistent with need, as when a person with pneumonia seeks medical treatment, but problems can arise when demand and need do not coincide. If individuals do not demand health services that medicine determines they need, it will lead to a worsening of their health and, for communicable diseases, that of others too. A persistent cough may not be recognized as a symptom of tuberculosis, leading to delayed diagnosis and risk of transmission. Needs may be less frequently translated into demand if services are not accessible, or if communities have a lower understanding of the potential for health intervention or low health literacy. When individuals demand health services that they do not need, resources are wasted and iatrogenesis may result, as when an individual experiences side effects from antibiotic treatment for a self-limiting respiratory illness caused by a virus infection. Demand from patients for a service can depend on the characteristics of the patient or on media and public interest in a service. Demand can also be induced by the supply of services. Geographical variation in hospital admission rates is explained more by the supply of hospital beds than by indicators of mortality; referral rates of general practitioners owe more to the characteristics of individual doctors than to the health of their populations (Wright et al., 1998).

'Supply' represents the willingness or ability of providers to deliver healthcare. It represents the total amount of healthcare available to consumers. The supply of healthcare depends on the interests of health professionals, the priorities of politicians, and the amount of resource available. The processes of needs assessment should aim to match the supply of services to population health needs. At the 'micro' level, where specific treatments are supplied to individual patients, research programmes for health technology assessment provide evidence concerning the clinical and cost effectiveness of new interventions. This evidence can be used to inform decisions on whether new interventions should be supplied by healthcare services through the deliberations of organizations like the National Institute for Health and Care Excellence (NICE) in the UK. At the 'meso' level of the healthcare organizational unit, and the 'macro' level of regional and national health systems, it is often more difficult to adopt an evidence-based approach. Normative and comparative metrics may be used to judge appropriate levels of supply in terms of numbers of primary care physicians or numbers of hospital beds per 1,000 population. When the total resources are well managed, the system creates openness in its capacity and ability to care for patients. Patients experience this openness primarily as the ability to access care without organizational barriers and with the timely availability of appointments with health and social care staff.

In the context of HCNA, the theoretical relationship between supply and demand has a practical application in adjusting the **capacity** to supply care against the **demand** expressed by consumers to the system. Analysing this relationship can create a shared understanding between providers and payers on demand, capacity, bottlenecks, and constraints, which can help to explain both the reasons why waiting lists grow and also the gap between the required capacity and the current capacity of a service. It can also help with modelling the required level of capacity to keep pace with demand (NHS England, 2019). Operational research techniques can be used to model patterns of demand and predictors of demands on services over time, so as to anticipate future levels of demands on services and the level of supply of services and staff required to meet these (NHS England, 2019).

6.8 What is a healthcare needs assessment?

Understanding the concept of need, and its relationship to supply and demand in healthcare, leads to an appreciation of how HCNA can be put to practical use in deploying services to improve population health. HCNA is

> a systematic process to assess the health problems facing a population. This includes determining whether certain groups appear more prone to illness than others and pinpointing any inequalities in terms of service provision. It results in an agreed list of priorities to improve healthcare in a particular area.
>
> **(National Institute for Health and Care Excellence, 2019)**

Wright described HCNA as using epidemiological, qualitative, and comparative methods to describe health problems of a population; to identify inequalities in health and access to services; and to determine priorities for the most effective use of resources (Wright et al., 1998; Williams & Wright, 1998). Williams and Wright (1998) described a 'triangle of health care needs assessment' (Figure 6.2) in which **epidemiological** data on the incidence and prevalence of diseases and other health conditions, together with health economic evidence on the **cost effectiveness** of services and other interventions, are mapped to a systematic description of **existing**

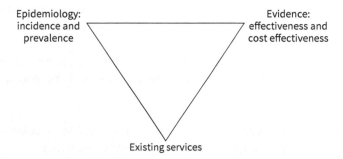

Figure 6.2 The triangulation of healthcare needs assessment

Adapted with permission from Wright et al. 'Epidemiological issues in health needs assessment.' *BMJ*, Vol. 316, Issue 7141, pp. 1379–82. Copyright © 1998 BMJ Publishing Group Ltd.

services to identify opportunities for change. This should raise crucial questions concerning whether existing services match the needs set out in the incidence or prevalence data, how gaps between population needs and existing services can be quantified, and what the most clinically and cost-effective means of addressing these gaps may be. This three-pronged approach should be kept in mind while undertaking the HCNA. HCNAs can become extremely complex, with multiple data sources and competing lines of activity and governance making it difficult to maintain the vision agreed at the outset. When this occurs, it is helpful to reframe the work undertaken in light of the three elements of the triangle, as this can help to navigate complexities and reset the vision.

6.9 Aims and objectives of healthcare needs assessment

Stevens and colleagues (2004) describe the overall aim of HCNA as being to 'provide information to plan, negotiate and change services for the better and to improve health in other ways'. In other words, the assessment can be performed with consideration for all activities that have an impact on health, whether directly in the hands of health services or not. The working definition of healthcare need as the population's ability to benefit from healthcare reflects this. The objectives are described by Stevens et al. (2004) as:

1. To specify services and other activities which impinge on healthcare—this is according to the triangle of HCNA.
2. Improving the spatial allocation of resources—this posits the notion of equity of access to services, with greater need leading to greater access to services, and equal need leading to equal access to services.
3. Target efficiency (i.e. the accurate targeting of resources to those in need), with the measurement of target efficiency being the measurement of whether or not, having assessed needs, resources are appropriately directed.
4. The gathering of general intelligence to get a perspective on population health and population health needs—this generally translates into the first practical step when undertaking a HCNA.
5. To stimulate the involvement and ownership of different players—the more that stakeholders are involved and the earlier they are involved, the more successful a HCNA is likely to be.

There are three key approaches to a HCNA, which can be used individually or in combination: epidemiological; corporate or qualitative; and comparative.

Needs assessment can be carried out at different levels including international, national, regional, local, and individual levels (Table 6.1) (Wilkinson & Murray, 1998).

Table 6.1 Levels for health needs assessment

Level	Population scale	Example
International	Billions	Global Burden of Disease Study; Disease Control Priorities in Developing Countries Report
National	Tens of Millions	Diabetes Prevention Programme
Regional	Millions	Liver transplantation
District level	Hundreds of thousands	Services for people with learning difficulties
General practice	Thousands	Services for infants and new mothers
Community or client group	Hundreds	Healthcare needs of new migrants, travellers, or homeless people
Individual	Individuals	Routine clinical practice

6.10 Epidemiological needs assessment

Epidemiological analysis is generally the first part of a HCNA that is undertaken, taking the form of an intensive intelligence-gathering exercise. The focus for the needs assessment should first be clearly specified through a precise and concise statement, often arrived at through consultation with stakeholders: for example, 'how can health services address the high mortality from breast cancer in this locality?' The focus for study should be supported by clear case definitions with agreed taxonomies for the categories and subcategories of conditions to be investigated. This requires awareness of the coding schemes that are in use in different sectors of healthcare. In the UK, the International Classification of Diseases, Tenth Revision is used for coding of hospital episode and mortality statistics, but the International Classification of Diseases for Oncology is used in the cancer registration system, while the Read code classification is used in primary care (though this is now being superseded by the Snomed classification). In the USA, the International Classification of Diseases, Ninth Revision, Clinical Modification (ICD-9-CM) is in wide use, while the Diagnostic and Statistical Manual of Mental Disorders (DSM-5) is employed by mental health services.

Epidemiological assessment should be undertaken with the help of specialists in public health data and intelligence who can provide access to epidemiological datasets concerning disease incidence, prevalence, and mortality, drawing on surveys, registries, and routine data sources. Data should be mapped to the three aspects of the needs assessment triangle. The greatest challenge will usually be to quantify the extent of unmet or unexpressed need. Here, it is important to specifically consider marginalized groups who may find existing services difficult to access, and may therefore be underenumerated in census data. Locally derived population-based estimates for incidence and prevalence may sometimes be available, as, for example, through the cancer registration system. More often, population-based data may be derived from national health surveys or registries developed in other localities. These data will be important for estimation of total need, including met and unmet need, but may not always be directly applicable to a particular locality.

Service mapping and process mapping have also become more important elements of HCNA, providing a detailed account of the supply of services and health service utilization. Analysis of health services data can contribute to service mapping, but health services data also contributes to epidemiological assessment of met need. This may include data concerning consultation and referral rates, screening rates, service access by locality, outcome data, and general practice register data for the prevalence of chronic diseases.

Descriptive epidemiological analysis traditionally emphasizes the attributes of variation by time, place, and person. Population data should be sourced to provide denominators for rates drawing on census data as well as population estimates and projections. Consideration should be given to age- and gender-specific estimates, in addition to age-standardized values, because local populations may have substantially different age distributions from those reported at national level. Trends over time can be evaluated graphically and through use of regression modelling. Use of geographical information system (GIS) software to facilitate mapping of epidemiological and health services utilization data may be very informative. Stratification by level of risk may also include levels of social and material deprivation or ethnic group.

Reports of well-designed evaluations and systematic reviews provide evidence of the effectiveness and cost effectiveness of potential interventions. In some instances, the report of a single randomized controlled trial might provide decisive evidence for a needs assessment. More often, a systematic review of all the well-designed studies on a given topic should be obtained or conducted. Guidelines from authoritative bodies at national level can also provide important evidence for cost-effective interventions and the appropriate design of care pathways (see Chapter 8 in this volume). More complex tools, such as programme budgeting and marginal analysis, can also be applied (as outlined in Chapter 10 in this volume).

6.11 Corporate needs assessment

The corporate approach to HCNA is where the demands, wishes, and alternative perspectives of key stakeholders are sourced and analysed. This part of the assessment may also provide an opportunity to identify key service-based datasets, such as clinic-based registers, which can be shared with the HCNA team. At the outset, it is wise to undertake a stakeholder mapping exercise. This is a dynamic process which should begin as an open-ended exercise, where the free flow of potential interest groups is discussed by the HCNA team. Subcategorization is a useful step here and includes, for example, members of the public, service users, service providers, commissioners, politicians, clinicians, and third-sector organizations. Lists of individuals who can be invited should be maintained. A stakeholder map can be produced based on the interests of different individuals and groups and their level of interest and influence.

The corporate element of a HCNA should ideally be undertaken as a **nested qualitative study** using recognized qualitative research methods including semi-structured interviews, and simple analysis and coding strategies to arrive at a list of major and recurrent themes. This adds a systematic level of methodology and allows structured analysis, lending legitimacy to the process and providing stakeholders with an opportunity to provide better considered responses. Corporate needs assessment may sometimes be used as the primary method of assessment, with the systematic collection of the knowledge and views of local health professionals and users of health services on healthcare services and needs (Adab et al., 2004). This allows the discovery of views on the perceived usefulness of proposed interventions and the preferences of patients and professionals who work with patients (Adab et al., 2004). Patients and members of the public represent an important stakeholder group who should have special representation and involvement in the HCNA process (as discussed in Chapter 4).

6.12 Comparative needs assessment

The comparative component of a needs assessment involves contrasting the services received by the population in one area to those in another, while taking into account differences between the populations in terms of demographic and socioeconomic measures. Reference can also be made to national benchmarks and other normative data. There are several ways of undertaking the comparative component of a needs assessment. A simple internet search can reveal other areas where similar HCNAs have been undertaken and structures, processes, and outcomes can be compared. To develop this further, there are a number of freely available tools such as those on the Public Health England Public Health Profiles (Public Health England, 2019) and a number of 'atlases' of data and outcomes that provide geographical comparison.

There are a number of sources of information for a comparative needs assessment. Some of the most straightforward data are health and social care activity data, and, where they are available, measures of health itself (such as incidence of specific diseases) should be used. In addition to comparing data from other areas, it may be useful to compare data with general practices serving the community in your area. Variations in activity between services may reveal important differences in health and social care practice. For example, effective clinical practice might be indicated by comparatively low numbers of prescriptions for sleeping tablets, tranquillizers, or antibiotics, and comparatively high numbers of prescriptions for antidepressants. For conditions such as asthma, good practice is thought to be indicated by a relatively high prescription rate of preventers (beclomethasone inhalers and similar) compared to symptom relievers (salbutamol inhalers and similar).

6.13 Strategic needs assessment

The concept of a 'strategic' health needs assessment first came to prominence in the UK in 2007, when the requirement for Joint Strategic Needs Assessment (JSNA) in the Local Government and Public Involvement in Health Act (2007) had the stated purpose of leading to stronger partnerships between communities, local government, and the NHS, providing a firm foundation for commissioning that improved health and social care provision and reduced inequalities. It was noteworthy that the word 'health' was removed, alluding to greater cooperation between primary care trusts (PCTs) and local authorities in the design, production, and governance of these reports. It was also stressed that JSNA was a process, not a product, and that iterative versions would be produced from year to year. JSNAs are now produced and updated on a regular basis throughout the country, and are designed to be used in a conjunction with Joint Health and Wellbeing Strategies, also produced by Health and Wellbeing Boards. Interestingly, there are examples of topic-specific strategic health needs assessments being used both as HCNAs and strategies (Bell, 2017).

6.14 Conclusions

It is important to consider that the audience for a HCNA may not be familiar with epidemiological and health economic techniques. It will also be important to produce reports and executive summaries that present the HCNA in an accessible manner, while presenting the underlying rationale for key conclusions. The findings of HCNAs will generally translate into a series of recommendations. These can be focused and service-specific, or they may be broader and more strategic. It is crucial that there should be a **clear line of sight** from evidence to recommendation.

At the broadest level, HCNAs can be considered to be instruments of change, facilitating transition from an undesirable state to one less undesirable/more desirable. Public health specialists sometimes complain that their carefully crafted HCNAs are left to 'sit on the shelf' after months of preparation, suggesting a waste of costly time and resources, and raising the question of whether it was the content or the distribution of the reports that was lacking. There are three key reasons why HCNAs may not be successful (Wright et al., 1998). Firstly, what is involved in assessing health needs and how it should be undertaken may not be understood. Starting with a simple and well-defined health topic can provide experience and encourage success. Secondly, there may be a lack of time, resources, or commitment. The time and resources required can be small when shared among professionals in a team, and such sharing has the potential to be team building. Integration of needs assessment into audit and education can also provide better use of scarce time. Such investment of time and effort is likely to become increasingly necessary in order to justify extra resources. Thirdly, results must be integrated with planning and purchasing intentions to ensure change. The planning cycle should begin with the assessment of need. Objectives must be clearly defined, and relevant stakeholders or agencies—be they primary care teams, hospital staff, health authorities, the voluntary sector, the media, regional executives, government, or patients—must be involved appropriately. Needs assessments that do not include sufficient attention to implementation will become little more than academic or public relations exercises.

The triangle of HCNA methodology also lends itself well to other evaluations such as service reviews, and although HCNAs have traditionally been undertaken by public health professionals looking at their local population, these local health needs should be paramount to all health professionals. Hospitals and primary care teams should both aim to develop services to match the needs of their local populations. Combining population needs assessment with personal knowledge of patients' needs may help to meet this goal (Wright et al., 1998).

References

Adab, P., et al. (2004). Use of a corporate needs assessment to define the information requirements of an arthritis resource centre in Birmingham: comparison of patients' and professionals' views. *Rheumatology*, 43(12), 1513–1518.

Barnett, K., Mercer, S.W., Norbury, M., Watt, G., Wyke, S., & Guthrie, B. (2012). Epidemiology of multimorbidity and implications for health care, research, and medical education: a cross-sectional study. *Lancet*, 380(9836), 37–43.

Bell, A. (2017). Meeting the need. What makes a 'good' JSNA for mental health or dementia? London: Centre for Mental Health. Available at: https://www.centreformentalhealth.org.uk/sites/default/files/2018-09/Centre_for_Mental_Health_Meeting_the_Need_JSNA.pdf [accessed 16 July 2019].

Bradshaw, J. (1972). Taxonomy of social need. In: In: G. McLachlan (ed.) *Problems and Progress in Medical Care: Essays on Current Research, 7th Series*. Oxford: Oxford University Press.

Culyer, A. (1998). Need–is a consensus possible? *J Med Ethics*, 24(2), 77–80.

Culyer, A.J. & Wagstaff, A. (1993). Equity and equality in health and health care. *J of Health Econ*, 12, 431–457.

Department of Health. (1989). *Working for Patients*. London: Department of Health.

Donaldson, C. & Mooney, G. (1991). Needs assessment, priority setting, and contracts for health care: an economic view. *BMJ (Clin Res)*, 303(6816), 1529–1530.

Hazra, N.C. & Gulliford, M. (2017). Evolution of the 'fourth stage' of epidemiologic transition in people aged 80 years and over: population-based cohort study using electronic health records. *Popul Health Metr*, 15, 10.

Local Government and Public Involvement in Health Act 2007 (Commencement No. 1 and Savings) Order. London: UK Parliament.

National Institute for Health and Care Excellence. (2019). *Health Needs Assessment*. London: NICE. Available at: https://www.nice.org.uk/glossary?letter=h.

NHS England. (2019). *About the Demand and Capacity Programme*. London: NHS England. Available at: https://www.england.nhs.uk/ourwork/demand-and-capacity/about/.

Public Health England. (2019). *Public Health Profiles*. London: Public Health England. Available at: https://fingertips.phe.org.uk/ [accessed 25 July 2019].

Stevens, A., Raftery, J., & Mant, J. (2004). The epidemiological approach to health care needs assessment. In: A. Stevens, J. Raftery, J. Mant, & S. Simpson (eds.) *Health Care Needs Assessment: The Epidemiologically Based Needs Assessment Reviews* (pp. 3–14). Oxford: Radcliffe Medical Press.

Tudor Hart, J. (2000). Commentary: three decades of the inverse care law. *BMJ*, 320(7226), 18–19.

Wilkinson, J.R. & Murray, S.A. (1998). Assessment in primary care: practical issues and possible approaches. *BMJ*, 316(7143), 1524.

Williams, R. & Wright, J. (1998). Epidemiological issues in health needs assessment. *BMJ (Clin Res)*, 316(7141), 1379–1382.

Wright, J., Williams, R., & Wilkinson, J.R. (1998). Development and importance of health needs assessment. *BMJ (Clin Res)*, 316(7140), 1310–1313.

7
Access to healthcare

Martin Gulliford

7.1 Introduction

'Access to healthcare' is concerned with the processes of gaining entry to the health-care system. One definition of access suggests that 'facilitating access is concerned with helping people to command appropriate health care resources in order to preserve or improve their health' (Gulliford et al., 2002). Access to healthcare is a complex concept that encompasses aspects of the ways that health services are financed, organized, and delivered, as well as the ways that different groups in the population interact with health services in order to obtain needed care. Figure 7.1 charts some of the key issues that contribute to access to healthcare and population coverage with health services. The chapter initially considers access to healthcare in a global context; it then discusses

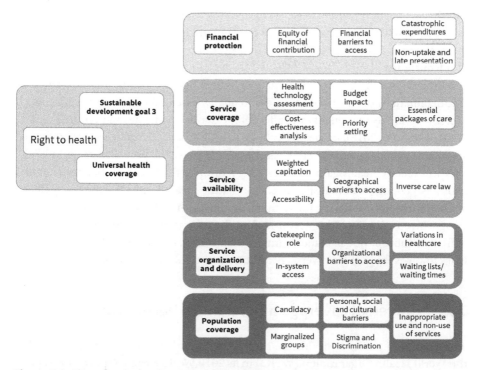

Figure 7.1 Map of some key issues in access to healthcare.

Martin Gulliford, *Access to healthcare* In: *Healthcare Public Health*. Edited by: Martin Gulliford and Edmund Jessop, Oxford University Press (2020). © Oxford University Press. DOI: 10.1093/oso/9780198837206.003.0007.

access at national and organizational levels, mainly focusing on high-income countries; in the final section of the chapter, access to healthcare is discussed from the perspective of service users. This discussion of access will touch briefly on many important issues in public health and health services: Is access to healthcare a human right? Does social justice require a fair distribution of health resources? How can fairness and equity of access be evaluated? Why do variations in healthcare develop and persist?

7.2 Access to healthcare in a global context

7.2.1 Access to healthcare as a human right

Healthcare has a special role in enabling people to live a full life span. Healthcare can reduce the impact of acute illnesses, minimize disability resulting from long-term conditions, and relieve pain and suffering at the end of life. All individuals have needs for healthcare over their life course. For these reasons, the United Nations (UN) recognized access to healthcare as a universal human right in the Universal Declaration of Human Rights of 1948 and the International Covenant on Economic, Social, and Cultural Rights (ICESCR) of 1966 (Office of the High Commissioner for Human Rights, 2019). Article 12 of the International Covenant recognizes 'the right of everyone to the enjoyment of the highest attainable standard of physical and mental health ... [including] all medical service and medical attention in the event of sickness' (Office of the High Commissioner for Human Rights, 2019). This legally binding international statement aims to ensure that all countries establish universal eligibility to adequate healthcare. This is reflected in the third UN Sustainable Development Goal (SDG) which includes the targets of 'achieving universal health coverage, including financial risk protection, access to quality essential health-care services and access to safe, effective, quality and affordable essential medicines and vaccines for all' (United Nations, 2018). In the SDG, access to healthcare and health service 'coverage' are almost synonymous. Coverage has been defined as 'the probability that individuals will receive health gain from an intervention if they need it' (Shengelia et al., 2005). No country can realistically claim that the ideal of universal access to all effective interventions is being fully achieved. Instead, the UN promotes the concept of 'progressive realisation'. This acknowledges the importance of resource constraints, which are more severe in some countries than others, but requires that all countries work towards the goal of universal healthcare over time (Hunt, 2007).

7.2.2 Universal coverage and financial barriers to access

The concept of access to healthcare as universal health coverage was developed by the World Health Organization (WHO) in its 2010 World Health Report. The Report identified three main dimensions of universal health coverage (Figure 7.2):

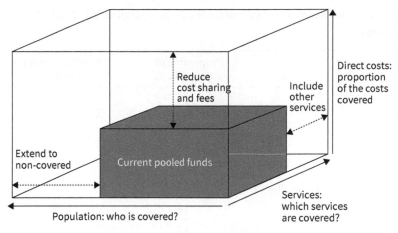

Three dimensions to consider when moving towards universal coverage

Figure 7.2 Three dimensions of universal health coverage.

Reproduced with permission from The World Health Organization (2010) 'Health systems financing: the path to universal coverage'. *World Health Report 2010*. Geneva: World Health Organization.

(i)   extending coverage of the population, so as to ensure that 'everyone who needs services should get them, not only those who can pay for them' (World Health Organization, 2010);

(ii) expanding the range of services covered, so that the quality of health services is sufficient to improve the health of the population; and

(iii) reducing financial risks through coverage of the costs of accessing healthcare.

This third dimension is critical to expanding health service coverage, but achieving this may require considerable political will because sharing the financial risks of healthcare implies a measure of commitment to social justice to enable those without resources to access healthcare. The need for healthcare arises unpredictably, the costs of accessing healthcare may be very high, and needs are generally greatest for those with fewest resources. Achieving universal health coverage requires that the 'healthy pay for services needed by the sick and the wealthy pay for services needed by the poor' (World Health Organization, 2010). However, this idea is not always politically and ideologically acceptable. Most high-income countries have embraced the ideal of universal health coverage, but the USA is an exception. In the UK, the National Health Service (NHS) was founded on the principles that it should meet the needs of everyone, that health services should be free at the point of delivery, and that eligibility for services should be based on clinical need, not ability to pay. These principles promote fairness or equity in terms of 'equal access for equal need'. This is sometimes referred to as the horizontal dimension of equity, which requires that equals should be treated equally.

Table 7.1 Global estimates of catastrophic health expenditures in 2010 (10% threshold)

	Proportion of population (%)	Number of people (million)
Global	11.7	808.4
Africa	11.4	118.7
Asia	12.8	531.1
Europe	7.2	53.2
Latin America and the Caribbean	14.8	88.3
North America	4.6	15.6
Oceania	3.9	1.4

Reproduced with permission from Wagstaff, A., et al. 'Progress on catastrophic health spending in 133 countries: a retrospective observational study'. *Lancet Glob Health*, Vol. 6, Issue 2, e169–e179. Copyright © 2018 Elsevier Inc.

Universal systems of healthcare, like the British NHS, remove most personal financial barriers to accessing health services, though even in Britain, prescription charges and transport costs to the health facility may impair access. This is not the case in most middle- and low-income countries, where a high proportion of all health service expenditures are out-of-pocket payments from service users to providers. The lack of affordability of health services for individuals and families is a key barrier to accessing healthcare. In these contexts, expenditures on healthcare represent a high proportion of household budgets, with financial impoverishment being exacerbated by loss of employment income through sickness. Health expenditures are labelled as 'catastrophic' when more than a specified proportion of annual household income is spent on healthcare. In a recent study, 11.7% of households globally, with 808 million people, incurred catastrophic health expenditures each year at the threshold of 10% of household income (Table 7.1). As expected, catastrophic expenditures were higher in countries with greater income inequality and lower government expenditures on healthcare (Wagstaff et al., 2018).

This analysis draws attention to equity in terms of the fairness of financial contribution to healthcare. One idea of social justice argues that, since poor health is largely a matter of misfortune at the individual level, if rational people view their prospects from behind a 'veil of ignorance' concerning their future health and social position, they will rationally choose an arrangement in which all individuals make a fair contribution to the costs, and receive a fair share of the benefits, of healthcare (Daniels, 2008; Rawls, 2007). The WHO 2010 Report on universal health coverage made a series of recommendations for achieving this objective.

7.3 Access to healthcare in the national context

7.3.1 Access as availability of health resources

In the national context, governments aim to facilitate access to healthcare by providing and commissioning health services. The question of how public healthcare resources should be allocated to different areas has been the subject of considerable study and debate. The historical pattern of supply of services is typically highly unequal, with more affluent urban areas having the greatest supply of services. In the UK, a resource allocation formula was developed with the aim of promoting the principle of equal access for equal need. Resources are allocated to local areas based on weighted capitation. The key element in the resource allocation formula is the size of the local population, but this is weighted for age to allow for the higher use of services by children and old people. The formula is also weighted for levels of population need. Estimation of healthcare needs is partly based on complex modelling of predictors of health service utilization, including level of deprivation. Unmet needs are incorporated using the standardized mortality ratio for the population under 75 years as an indicator of unmet need. Resource allocation formulae also allow for the varying supply costs of delivering care in different areas. There is evidence of an ecological association between changes in healthcare resource allocation over time and changes in mortality amenable to healthcare intervention (Barr et al., 2014). Implementation of the weighted capitation formula resulted in a more rapid increase in healthcare funding in deprived areas, and this was associated with more rapid declines in mortality amenable to healthcare interventions in these areas, though mortality remained substantially higher in association with deprivation (Barr et al., 2014).

7.3.2 Service coverage and priority setting

As well as determining how healthcare resources should be allocated, national governments may contribute to establishing procedures to determine how healthcare resources should utilized. Over the last two decades, there has been a drive to improve the efficiency and effectiveness of health services by promoting evidence-based healthcare. This encourages healthcare practices based on well-designed research studies that provide evidence of the effectiveness of health interventions, with clinical trials and meta-analyses of clinical trials considered to represent the highest levels of evidence. The opportunity cost of delivering ineffective procedures is represented by the effective treatments that cannot be delivered because of lack of resources. Since it is often difficult to disinvest from ineffective procedures that are already in widespread use, it is important to ensure that evaluation is performed before new health technologies are introduced.

The UK government established a programme of applied health research, through the National Institute of Health Research, with a significant focus on health technology assessment. Health economic evaluations, alongside clinical trials, have provided evidence of cost effectiveness that employs generic metrics, such as the cost per quality adjusted life year (QALY), that can be compared across different clinical interventions. In England and Wales, the government established the National Institute for Health and Care Excellence (NICE), with a role in evaluating the evidence to support new and existing health technologies and proving guidance on their utilization. NICE generally employs a threshold value of £20,000 to £30,000 per QALY to determine whether a technology provides value for money and should be offered in the NHS. The requirement for evaluation, and the use of cost-effectiveness thresholds, might sometimes disadvantage patients with rare diseases or very short life expectancy because treatments for these groups might often be costly to develop, and evidence of effectiveness might be more difficult to demonstrate. In response to public concerns, the UK government set up a special 'cancer drugs fund' to enable patients with advanced cancer to access new drug treatments, which may be very costly. However, this has proved controversial and difficult to justify in terms of value for money.

The question of the affordability of health interventions is now being considered at the health-system level. In the UK, affordability of new services is currently evaluated not only in terms of cost effectiveness but also in terms of the overall budgetary impact of a new intervention, with interventions having a budgetary impact of more than £20 million per year in England being subject to further negotiation (Charlton et al., 2017). In low-income countries, the World Bank proposed that limited government health resources should be invested in 'essential packages of care' that only include highly cost-effective interventions of low budget impact. This approach though has proved difficult to implement in practice (World Health Organization, 2013)

In the UK, local areas may have considerable discretion over the services that are selected for funding. This can lead to wide variations in service provision, with novel interventions such as high-cost cancer drugs being available in some areas but not others. This is sometimes referred to as a 'postcode lottery' because of the inconsistency arising from the horizontal equity principle. This highlights a growing debate concerning the ethical principles that should be employed in priority setting and the procedures that should be used to deliver these (Norheim, 2016). The WHO encourages the use of cost-effectiveness analysis in priority setting, with a broadly utilitarian approach of promoting efficiency and maximizing aggregate benefits. At the same time, affirmation of the 'right to health' might require that certain individuals should receive a share of healthcare in the interests of fairness, even though this might diminish the overall sum of health gains (Norheim, 2016; Daniels, 2008). As well as achieving fair outcomes, fair and transparent processes should be employed to reach decisions of this nature. Trade-offs between equity and efficiency should be established in a transparent and consistent way, with engagement of the public, in order to ensure that decision-making bodies show accountability for the reasonableness of their priority-setting and resource-allocation decisions (Daniels, 2008).

7.3.3 Access as availability of services

In the absence of regulation, health services tend to be better developed in more affluent areas of population concentration: areas where it is pleasant to live and where prospective patients can pay doctors' fees. The British general practitioner Julian Tudor Hart coined the term 'inverse care law' to describe this state of affairs where 'the availability of good medical care tends to vary inversely with the need for it in the population served' (Tudor Hart, 1971). There is ample evidence to support this 'law': deprived inner-city areas with poor health metrics generally have a lower supply of primary care physicians per 1,000 population. In less densely populated rural areas, problems of service availability relate less to the absolute level of supply than to distances and travel times from service providers. There is often evidence for a decay effect, with utilization decreasing with increasing distance from the provider location (Kelly et al., 2016). Specialist services often achieve better outcomes when they are concentrated at centres with higher volumes of work, but spatial equity can be promoted through satellite clinics and utilization of electronic media for communication with patients and remote sites.

7.3.4 Access as utilization of health resources

Donabedian (1972) argued that utilization of health services is the proof of access to healthcare. Access based on utilization of healthcare may be evaluated both in terms of 'entry' access, which concerns initial contacts with the healthcare system, and 'in-system' access, which concerns patients' progression between different levels of care once entry access has been achieved. In the UK, and in other countries with better-developed systems of primary care, general practitioners (GPs) and primary care physicians have a 'gatekeeping role' in which they regulate access to specialist and hospital care. This is important in ensuring efficient use of healthcare resources. GPs generally operate in an environment where more serious diagnoses are infrequent and tests have low predictive values. Specialists are accustomed to working in a context where serious abnormalities are common and test predictive values are high. Consequently, allowing direct access to specialist care by the general population may lead to overinvestigation and overtreatment. However, the gatekeeping function can perpetuate or exacerbate inequalities in access if better-educated, higher-income groups are able to negotiate better access to specialist care. A broadly consistent finding from studies to date is that lower socioeconomic groups tend to be higher users of primary care and emergency services, but the same groups show lower uptake of preventive medical interventions and specialist care (Dixon–Woods et al., 2006). In a study of health systems in the Organization for Economic and Co-operative Development (OECD), van Doorslaer and colleagues (2006) found that after adjusting for needs, lower-income groups generally showed similar utilization of primary care services than higher-income groups but, in most countries, there was evidence of pro-rich inequity in the utilization of specialist physician visits. The magnitude of these inequalities varied across health systems, with those systems relying on private insurance or out-of-pocket payments generally showing larger differences by income level.

Waiting times and delays in treatment may also be indicative of problems of 'in-system' access and organizational barriers to care. These problems may result from a mismatch of supply and demand for services, but may also result from inefficient use of existing capacity in terms of scheduling of appointments or use of day-case services. These organizational barriers may impact on the timeliness of care delivery, which may be important for the prognosis of some conditions such as cancer.

7.3.5 Variations in services

As well as showing systematic variation according to deprivation or socioeconomic level, there are wide, seemingly random, variations in the utilization of health services in different areas. Wennberg and Gittelsohn (1973) showed that the numbers of common surgical procedures varied widely in different areas within the American state of Vermont. The variation was highest for tonsillectomy, with a 12-fold difference in rates between areas, but other procedures such as hernia repair, cholecystectomy, and hysterectomy varied between two- and five-fold. Medical practice variations have been confirmed by many studies reported from different contexts, with wide variations demonstrated in international comparative studies. These variations in utilization suggest that there are wide variations in access to healthcare. However, variations appear to arise when there is a lack of clear evidence of effectiveness, leading to wide clinical discretion in the decision to use specific procedures. Clinicians may form differing views on the indications for surgery, and patients may also form their own preferences as to whether surgery is used or not. For example, patients with early stage prostate cancer might reasonably be offered a choice between surgical treatment and 'watchful waiting' because the benefits and harms of early intervention may be valued differently by different patients. In addition, the health system may offer incentives that influence the use of surgery such as distances to be travelled, the method of payment, and regulatory factors that influence the uptake of new procedures (Birkmeyer et al., 2013).

Variations also exist in the delivery of most aspects of primary care services (Figure 7.3). This may apply to aspects that are associated with considerable clinical and provider discretion, such as hospital referrals. There is also variation in the delivery of evidence-based care for long-term conditions like diabetes and asthma with lack of achievement of key measures of process of care and intermediate outcomes such as risk factor control. This means that there are inequalities in patients' access to effective management for these conditions. In recent years, there have been considerable efforts directed at quality improvement, including mandatory continuing professional

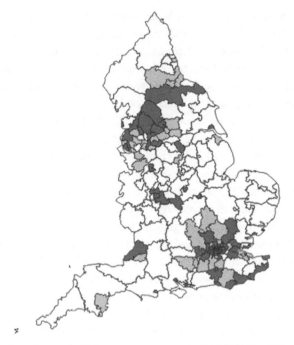

Figure 7.3 Variations in access to breast cancer screening in England. Dark grey areas have lower screening rates; white areas, higher screening rates; medium grey areas are similar to the national average.

Reproduced from Public Health England (2019). *Public Health Profiles*. London: Public Health England. Available at https://fingertips.phe.org.uk/

updating and audit. In England, the government introduced a financial incentive scheme known as the 'Quality and Outcomes Framework' (QOF) which rewards general practices for achieving specified standards of chronic illness care for their re-gistered patients. The implementation of this scheme was shown to reduce inequal-ities in service delivery in primary care across a range of tracer conditions (Doran et al., 2008).

7.4 The service user perspective and barriers to access

Up to this point, access to healthcare has mainly been considered from the health system provider perspective. In an early analysis, Pechansky and Thomas (1981) char-acterized the concept of 'access' as representing the 'degree of fit' between the patient and the healthcare system. This draws attention to the importance of service users' perspectives in defining access. Some writers view potential patients as negotiating a series of barriers to accessing care. These include financial barriers related to the affordability of services, geographical barriers related to service accessibility, and organizational barriers related to methods of organizing care that may have the effect of restricting access and utilization. Personal, social, and cultural barriers to accessing care are also important in influencing whether services can be utilized, even when these are available. Barriers to access increase the amount of 'work' that patients have to do to gain access to healthcare (Dixon–Woods et al., 2006). Such barriers typically represent more severe obstacles for some groups in the population.

Membership of minority social groups or living in poverty can lead to exclusion from many social activities including engagement with healthcare services. Socially excluded groups may include new migrants, travellers, homeless people, prisoners, people with serious mental illness, and members of ethnic minority groups, to name but a few. These groups are sometimes referred to as 'hard to reach', but this is now regarded as an inappropriate term and a more neutral terminology of 'marginalized' groups is recommended. Members of marginalized groups may experience unusual difficulties in gaining access to healthcare for a variety of reasons including lack of a fixed address, language difficulties, lack of education, and low health literacy. Membership of a marginalized group may be associated with stigma and negative stereotyping; stigmatized conditions including substance abuse, mental health disorders, and infections may be more frequent in these groups. Public health action at the local level requires assessing the needs of people in socially excluded groups, taking steps to address barriers to access, and designing services that are responsive and acceptable. For example, outreach services may make special efforts to engage with underserved groups. These actions help to promote equity in its vertical dimension, ensuring that unequals are treated in proportion to their inequality. Relying on the principle of equal access for equal need may not be sufficient to ensure fair treatment of marginalized groups because their needs may be qualitatively different from those of the majority.

Barriers to access may contribute to non-use of needed services, resulting in reduced coverage of effective interventions. However, apparently 'inappropriate' use of services may also be indicative of access problems, reflecting a lack of fit between user wants and demands and service providers' expectations. Dixon–Woods and colleagues (2006) suggested that access to services should be interpreted in terms of 'candidacy', with the notion that people's eligibility for healthcare is jointly negotiated between themselves and health services. Both health services and potential service users are constantly revising their ideas about what conditions represent appropriate circumstances for medical intervention. Consequently, it is not surprising that expectations may sometimes be mismatched, nor that this mismatch may be greatest for lower socioeconomic and marginalized groups.

The principle of fairness requires that access to healthcare does not depend on individual characteristics such as age, gender, ethnic group, or sexual orientation. There is much evidence to show that, in reality, health service utilization is often strongly patterned by these characteristics. It may not always be easy to determine whether this differential use of health services results from real variations in patients' needs or from covert discrimination against certain groups of service users. This concern is particularly relevant for the rapidly growing population of older adults. The ageing population is often cited as a driver of increasing healthcare costs but recent analyses showed that, after allowing for proximity to death, healthcare costs may actually diminish at advanced ages (Hazra et al., 2017). Less intensive treatment of older adults might reflect patients' preferences but might also reflect an implied lower priority for treatment at older ages. This was suggested by Alan Williams as the 'fair innings' argument, where treatment could ethically be considered lower priority after a fair life span, perhaps 70 years, had been achieved (Hazra et al., 2018). This approach appears to have some measure of public support, but is difficult to justify on ethical and practical grounds (Hazra et al., 2018). The English NHS has now developed an ethical framework which requires that decisions at the priority-setting level should only be based on clinical need: services 'should not give preferential treatment to any individual patients who are one of a group of patients with the same clinical needs'(National Health Service, 2013).

7.5 Evaluating access at health-service level

The multidimensional nature of access to healthcare is exemplified in developments in cancer services in the UK. Several studies showed that cancer survival in the UK was generally lower than in comparator countries in Europe (Berrino et al., 2007). This led to multiple streams of service development, supported by research, to increase access to effective cancer care and improve cancer outcomes. Peoples' reluctance to enter a pathway that may lead to cancer diagnosis represents a barrier to early cancer detection. This was addressed through public mass media campaigns encouraging people to consult a doctor if they had 'alarm symptoms' suggestive of cancer, thus promoting early 'entry' access. GPs were encouraged to ensure early referral to specialist services of patients who might have cancer. A 'two-week wait' referral process was established to overcome organizational barriers and ensure that rapid 'in-system' access was established (Møller et al., 2015). Organizational barriers to accessing cancer care were addressed by establishing cancer networks, to ensure that all patients with cancer were treated by clinicians who were expert in the management of a specific cancer type. Multidisciplinary teams were set up to ensure that all patients had access to the most effective specialist treatment options including surgery, radiotherapy, and chemotherapy. Resources were allocated to new radiotherapy treatment facilities, in order to reduce waiting times, as well as to new drug treatments. Efforts are being made to ensure that all eligible patients receive high-quality palliative care, wherever they live. These developments combine to ensure that 'access' is enabled across the entire cancer-treatment pathway.

7.6 Conclusion

Maxwell suggested that there are six dimensions for health service evaluation: access, equity, effectiveness, efficiency, acceptability, and relevance to need (Maxwell, 1984).

These dimensions are closely interrelated. This chapter has focused on the dimension of access to healthcare, but this has been seen to be closely related to the concept of equity. Considerations of effectiveness and efficiency have been seen to be of importance on the provider side, while acceptability and relevance to need are important to service users. There have been many attempts to evaluate the overall performance of health systems, and evaluation of access is a key element of almost all of these (Braithwaite et al., 2017).

In its 2017 comparison of 11 health systems, the American Commonwealth Fund employed indicators on five domains, with access and equity included as main domains. Information about access was derived from survey respondents concerning the affordability and timeliness of care, while the equity domain comprised a comparison of other domain indicators across low- and high-income levels. The results of the Commonwealth Fund analysis suggested that national health systems funded through general taxation of national health insurance (UK, Australia, Netherlands) generally score higher on access and equity than systems that rely on private health insurance (Canada, France, USA). An essential health service coverage index was developed using data for 16 tracer conditions (Hogan et al., 2018). Analysis of this new index suggested that the goals of universal health coverage have largely been achieved in many high-income countries including the UK and Western Europe (see Figure 7.2). In low-income countries, severe resource constraints limit the achievement of universal health coverage.

References

Barr, B., Bambra, C., & Whitehead, M. (2014). The impact of NHS resource allocation policy on health inequalities in England 2001–11: longitudinal ecological study. *BMJ*, 348, g3231.

Berrino, F., et al. (2007). Survival for eight major cancers and all cancers combined for European adults diagnosed in 1995–99: results of the EUROCARE-4 study. *Lancet Oncol*, 8, 773–783.

Birkmeyer, J.D., Reames, B.N., McCulloch, P., Carr, A.J., Campbell, W.B., & Wennberg, J.E. (2013). Understanding of regional variation in the use of surgery. *Lancet*, 382, 1121–1129.

Braithwaite, J., et al. (2017). Health system frameworks and performance indicators in eight countries: a comparative international analysis. *SAGE Open Med*, 5, 2050312116686516.

Charlton, V., et al. (2017). Cost effective but unaffordable: an emerging challenge for health systems. *BMJ*, 356, j1402.

Daniels, N. (2008). *Just Health*. Cambridge: Cambridge University Press.

Dixon–Woods, M., et al. (2006). Conducting a critical interpretive synthesis of the literature on access to health care by vulnerable groups. *BMC Med Res Methodol*, 6, 35.

Donabedian, A. (1972). Models for organising the delivery of personal health services and criteria for evaluating them. *Milbank Mem Fund Quart*, 50, 103–154.

Doran, T., Fullwood, C., Kontopantelis, E., & Reeves, D. (2008). Effect of financial incentives on inequalities in the delivery of primary clinical care in England: analysis of clinical activity indicators for the quality and outcomes framework. *Lancet*, 372, 728–736.

Gulliford, M., et al. (2002). What does 'access to health care' mean? *J Health Serv Res Policy*, 7, 186–188.

Hazra, N.C., Gulliford, M.C., & Rudisill, C. (2018). 'Fair innings' in the face of ageing and demographic change. *Health Econ Policy Law,* 13, 209–217.

Hazra, N.C., Rudisill, C., & Gulliford, M.C. (2017). Determinants of health care costs in the senior elderly: age, comorbidity, impairment, or proximity to death? *Eur J Health Econ.* 19, 831–842.

Hogan, D.R., Stevens, G.A., Hosseinpoor, A.R., & Boerma, T. (2018). Monitoring universal health coverage within the Sustainable Development Goals: development and baseline data for an index of essential health services. *Lancet Glob Health,* 6, e152–e168.

Hunt, P. (2007). Right to the highest attainable standard of health. *Lancet,* 370, 369–371.

Kelly, C., Hulme, C., Farragher, T., & Clarke, G. (2016). Are differences in travel time or distance to health care for adults in global north countries associated with an impact on health outcomes? A systematic review. *BMJ Open,* 6, e013059.

Maxwell, R.J. (1984). Quality assessment in health. *BMJ (Clin Res Ed),* 288, 1470–1472.

Møller, H., Gildea, C., Meechan, D., Rubin, G., Round, T., & Vedsted, P. (2015). Use of the English urgent referral pathway for suspected cancer and mortality in patients with cancer: cohort study. *BMJ,* 351, h5102.

National Health Service. (2013). *Commissioning Policy: Ethical Framework for Priority Setting and Resource Allocation.* London: Department of Health. Available at: https://www.england. nhs.uk/wp-content/uploads/2013/04/cp-01.pdf [accessed 16 July 2019].

Norheim, O.F. (2016). Ethical priority setting for universal health coverage: challenges in deciding upon fair distribution of health services. *BMC Med,* 14, 75.

Office of the High Commissioner for Human Rights. (2019). *International Covenant on Economic, Social and Cultural rights.* Geneva: Office of the High Commissioner for Human Rights. Available at: https://www.ohchr.org/en/professionalinterest/pages/cescr.aspx [accessed 16 July 2019].

Pechansky, R. & Thomas, W. (1981). The concept of access. *Med Care,* 19, 127–140.

Public Health England. (2019). *Public Health Profiles.* London: Public Health England. Available at https://fingertips.phe.org.uk/ [accessed 25 July 2019].

Rawls, J. (2007). *Theory of Justice.* Harvard: Harvard University Press.

Shengelia, B., Tandon, A., Adams, O.B., & Murray, C.J.L. (2005). Access, utilization, quality, and effective coverage: an integrated conceptual framework and measurement strategy. *Soc Sci Med,* 61, 97–109.

Tudor Hart, J. (1971). The inverse care law. *Lancet,* 1(7696), 405–412.

United Nations. (2018). *Sustainable Development Goals.* New York: United Nations. Available at: https://www.un.org/sustainabledevelopment/sustainable-development-goals/ [accessed 16 July 2019].

van Doorslaer, E., Masseria, C., Koolman, X., & for the OECD Health Equity Research Group. (2006). Inequalities in access to medical care by income in developed countries. *CMAJ,* 174(2), 177–183.

Wagstaff, A., et al. (2018). Progress on catastrophic health spending in 133 countries: a retrospective observational study. *Lancet Glob Health,* 6, e169–e179.

Wennberg, J. & Gittelsohn, A. (1973). Small area variations in health care delivery. *Science,* 182(4117), 1102–1108.

World Health Organization. (2010). *Health Systems Financing: The Path to Universal Coverage. World Health Report 2010.* Geneva: World Health Organization.

World Health Organization. (2013). *Essential Health Service Packages.* Geneva: World Health Organization.

8
Knowledge management
Evidence into guidance

Aoife Molloy

8.1 Introduction: the role of evidence

Research is continuously generating new evidence at an increasing rate. This new evidence offers the potential for improvements and advances in healthcare. Evidence may include new knowledge from basic sciences, patient-centred clinical studies, epidemiological analyses, behavioural science research, health economics, and health systems' research to inform the design and delivery of healthcare. New evidence may help to tackle complex and challenging clinical scenarios, tailor treatment plans for individuals, provide the highest value care, and ensure good stewardship of resources, as well as inform the optimal organization and delivery of services. We can use evidence to address all aspects of healthcare including diagnostic dilemmas, treatment decisions, health promotion, prevention of disease, design of care settings, safe staffing levels and appropriate task allocation, national and local healthcare resource allocation, and patient involvement and engagement in all aspects of healthcare. Despite the growing body of evidence, improvements in healthcare quality are not guaranteed. Evidence must be interpreted, translated into practice, and the impact measured. For this to be achieved, evidence generation and evidence synthesis must address relevant questions and tackle the important challenges facing healthcare services around the world.

In a global context, health systems face the challenges of increasing longevity, growing complexity of healthcare needs, emerging new technologies and treatments, the growing prevalence of long-term conditions, and the importance of inequalities in health and healthcare access. There are also difficulties of ensuring that health services provide integrated and coordinated care, with fragmentation of care being a common problem. We need to ensure that knowledge management addresses these issues and does not contribute to them by focusing on single conditions and diseases, without regard to the rising prevalence of multimorbidity. Knowledge management should be used to guide more coherent care across healthcare systems. Evidence and knowledge management must also promote appropriateness in healthcare. As complexity of treatment and disease increases, delivery of healthcare is becoming increasingly multidisciplinary and patient-centred. Knowledge management should guide careful use of resources. As

Aoife Molloy, *Knowledge management* In: *Healthcare Public Health*. Edited by: Martin Gulliford and Edmund Jessop,
Oxford University Press (2020). © Oxford University Press. DOI: 10.1093/oso/9780198837206.003.0008.

science advances, so too must ethical discussion of the limits and risks of health-care interventions.

8.2 Applying evidence to care

The evidence base of research studies with the potential to inform healthcare organization and delivery is vast, but this cannot be readily implemented by individuals or healthcare provider organizations. Evidence must first be quality assured, interpreted, and summarized. Knowledge management and guidance development address this need. Managing knowledge and evidence to develop guidance to improve healthcare quality must be a rigorous, pragmatic, transparent, and trusted process. Guidance encompasses recommendations developed through systematic knowledge management. It aims to improve the quality and safety of healthcare by systematically synthesizing and appraising available evidence and providing consensus expert opinion when evidence is lacking or inconclusive. Guidance establishes best practice and can reduce unwarranted variation and inequality. The term 'guidelines' encompasses clinical practice guidelines as well as guidelines addressing broader topics including public health and health-service design and delivery. Clinical practice guidelines generally present recommendations on how to diagnose and treat a medical condition, but guidelines on broader health-system processes have been developed, including guidance on safe staffing levels or workplace health-management practices.

Knowledge management enables the processes of evidence identification, synthesis, and appraisal to be centralized. A centralized approach offers efficiencies of scale, including access to multidisciplinary expert advisers, pooled resources, and development of more rigorous and tested approaches. This generally permits a higher standard of analysis with the opportunity to develop national consensus. However, centralized guidance development may be remote from the end users, and consideration must be given to broad dissemination strategies. Consultation that invites and engages with a diverse population of service providers and users is also important in ensuring that guidance addresses key concerns, including ethical issues such as fairness. Plans for the implementation and mobilization of resources, as well as for evaluation of the impact of evidence, can be made on a large scale, thus achieving a higher impact.

8.3 Topic selection and question development

The topic of a guideline defines the subject area on which the guideline will focus questions. Ministries of health or other national organizations can propose topics to guideline developers. In England, NHS England, the Department of Health and Social Care, and Public Health England refer topics to the National Institute for Health and Care Excellence (NICE) for development into guidelines. Members of the public, patients, clinicians, and other individuals or organizations in the healthcare system can also suggest topics. Topics must address relevant issues faced in healthcare. Specialist societies may address topics that are suggested by their members. Guideline development requires investment of resources and time. Guideline-producing organizations can be commissioned to focus on a specific topic, and from this must develop the question addressed by the guidance and the scope of the guidance.

Importantly, the scope of the guidance defines what it will and will not focus on, and predetermines the recommendations' impact and rigour. The scope also identifies the population that the guidance will cover, and the key questions concerning both clinical and cost effectiveness that will be addressed. The scope must be clear and agreed before evidence identification and appraisal, as it will determine the questions asked for the literature reviews.

The review questions inform the literature search strategy. They can examine causal relationships, associations, impact of interventions, settings where interventions work best, technologies, treatments, views of service users and healthcare practitioners, resource impact, and unintended consequences. Several frameworks can be used to structure the review questions to ensure all aspects of the query are examined: for example, PICO (population, intervention, comparators, outcome) or SPICE (setting, perspective, intervention, comparison, evaluation) (World Health Organization, 2012; NICE, 2014).

8.4 Sources of evidence

Evidence identification, appraisal, and synthesis are key components of knowledge management and guideline development. Literature searches should be reproducible, systematic, and transparently documented, with clear inclusion and exclusion criteria that identify the best evidence to answer the guideline question. The databases selected for searching and the types of evidence sought may vary depending on the subject area of the guideline. The quality of evidence depends on the designs of included studies, the endpoints selected for evaluation, as well as other aspects of study design that affect the risk of bias. Evidence is ranked at different levels indicating its relative strength, from the lowest, potentially most biased (expert opinion), to higher levels with a lower risk of bias (randomized controlled trials and meta-analyses). The level of evidence is embodied in the selection criteria for a review in terms of the eligible designs. Selecting a higher level of evidence aims to reduce the risk of bias but does not guarantee the quality of the research.

Evidence from clinical trials, population-based cohort studies, qualitative studies, registries, and, increasingly, real-world data can inform guideline recommendations (Williams et al., 2019). Information on patient perspectives and experiences can be identified from these sources, but broader and richer information may be obtained from patient-reported outcomes measures (PROMs) and patient-reported experience measures (PREMs). PROMS and PREMS are validated instruments used to measure, for example, self-reported health status, functional ability, and perception of experience of care (Kingsley & Patel, 2017). Real-world data (RWD), in the form of routinely collected administrative electronic health records, are used progressively to generate real-world evidence (RWE). RWE may help to address gaps in evidence and answer guideline questions: for example, for those people who are not traditionally enrolled in clinical trials due to extremes of age or to complexity of multiple or rare long-term conditions (Hernan & Robins, 2016).

Currently, selection bias and a lack of comparator data, together with a scarcity of statistical capabilities to overcome these limitations, hamper RWE application. Comparative effectiveness research (CER) may help to solve the problem of lacking comparator data and answer questions about benefits of interventions in a real-world setting. CER compares different interventions using the same health-based outcomes to inform which interventions offer the most value in a population. The Observational Medical Outcomes Partnership (OMOP) Common Data Model allows systematic analysis of different datasets by transforming data (often from electronic health records) into a common format. It provides an example of CER that uses RWD to address gaps in evidence (Ogunyemi et al., 2013).

The aforementioned evidence sources provide information on the efficacy and effectiveness of interventions. The efficacy of an intervention relates to whether it produces the intended result in controlled settings. The effectiveness of an intervention, on the other hand, is concerned with how well the intervention produces the intended result in usual, everyday settings, where variables and patient characteristics cannot be controlled. The external validity of some trials is limited and so the results may not be readily applied in wider contexts. The intended outcomes are influenced in clinical practice by the doctor–patient relationship, placebo effects, and patient preference (Rothwell, 2005).

Observational data are particularly used to evaluate safety outcomes because of the lower risk of confounding by indication for these outcomes (Vandenbroucke, 2004). Information from safety alert systems—for example, the Medicines and Healthcare Regulatory Agency (MHRA) yellow card scheme used to report adverse effects of medical products, and the National Reporting and Learning System (NRLS) used to report safety incidents in healthcare—is also used to inform guideline development.

Economic analyses form a significant component of the evidence examined in knowledge management and guideline development. Recommendations are informed by evidence of effectiveness of an intervention. The cost effectiveness of interventions is often included in the effectiveness analysis, considering the question of what outcomes can be expected and at what cost. Quality adjusted life years (QALYs) are used as summary measures of the value of an intervention based on patient-reported changes in health-related quality of life. These measures allow comparison of different interventions and the impact of the interventions for different people with different illnesses.

The relative cost effectiveness of health interventions may be compared using incremental cost-effectiveness ratios (ICERs), which incorporate the incremental outcomes and costs of different interventions. New interventions should be compared with current best practice (the comparator) in a randomized trial to inform an economic analysis. In the absence of trial data, it may be challenging to attribute changes in outcomes to interventions, and as such, evidence of effectiveness may sometimes be lacking. To support the development of clear recommendations for guidelines, economic models are used to predict the impact of the intervention on the broader health system or pathway. Modelling helps to consider the benefits of interventions as well as the unintended consequences, and the opportunity cost (NICE, 2014).

The guideline committee must then consider the economic analysis to understand the cost of an intervention in relation to the gains for a patient or population. However, decisions should not be made on cost-effectiveness analysis alone because this only represents one ethical viewpoint—the utilitarian ideal of the 'greatest good for the greatest number'. To make recommendations and influence population health impact and spending, the guideline committee must apply social value judgements while appraising evidence of effectiveness. Recommendations on smoking bans may infringe on an individual's right to individual choice but benefit the population as a whole. Social value judgements take into account cultural, ethical, and population-wide considerations to recommend what is best for society (Shah et al., 2013).

8.5 Grading guidelines

The process of evidence synthesis must be transparent and must follow accepted methodology. The quality of the evidence should be graded using internationally recognized instruments. Systematic reviews are used in guideline development to address predetermined questions and include all empirical evidence that address the questions asked and meet predefined criteria. Meta-analysis is used to summarize the results of a systematic review using statistical methods.

The strength of the evidence used in guideline development and the quality of the developed recommendations must be appraised and clearly stated. Evidence and recommendations can be graded separately or together, using recognized tools. Internationally recognized instruments such as GRADE are widely used and allow appraisal of the strength of the evidence and the quality of the recommendations that are developed from it (Guyatt et al., 2008).

Transparent processes for development of guidelines, following accepted methodology with rigorous evidence appraisal and grading of recommendations, should be used. Guideline methodology evaluated by international organizations such as the Guidelines International Network (G-I-N) should be followed in a diligent and transparent fashion, and methods should be reviewed using instruments such as AGREE II (Brouwers et al., 2016).

8.6 Limitations of evidence

Despite the vast evidence available, knowledge management and quality improvement may be hampered by the limitations or lack of availability of evidence to address key guideline questions. The complexity of real clinical scenarios is poorly captured in research studies. The growing population of older people with multimorbidity is also poorly served by guidance that is based on evidence focusing on single conditions (Hughes et al., 2013). Important drug interactions and overinvestigation may occur. Clinical trial data for subgroups (for example, older people or those with multimorbidity) are often limited in sample size. Long-term follow-up data are not always available, and so recommendations have to be developed through expert consensus. Increasingly, RWD and RWE are being employed to address the limitations of traditional sources of information. For example, NICE used RWD from the National Joint Registry for England and Wales on type of hip prosthesis and time to revision, to inform decision making, as data from clinical trials were lacking. However, NICE guidance did not recommend a particular hip prosthesis (Bell et al., 2016).

8.7 Decision making

Expert opinion and consensus are necessary to develop recommendations. Gaps in the evidence and conflicting, incomplete, or poor-quality evidence or lack of evidence that is applicable to the guideline question often result in confusion and variation in the delivery of healthcare. This is where guidelines can offer value. Guideline committees or development groups appraise evidence and can make carefully weighted and informed recommendations where there is ambiguity or uncertainty (Wieringa et al., 2018). Formal consensus techniques—for example, the Delphi Method or the RAND/ UCLA Appropriateness Method—are sometimes used to provide a framework for group decision making (Lawson et al., 2012).

Guidance recommendations informed by evidence and developed using social value judgements form the basis for how the guideline will be implemented and the impact it will have. In developing recommendations, the guideline committee should consider the implications on current practice, innovation, variation, and equality and recommend a gold standard that is achievable. The use of clear and unambiguous language is essential (World Health Organization, 2012; NICE, 2014).

Successful implementation of guidance depends, in part, on how it is tailored to the audience. Guidance should be relevant to multidisciplinary teams, but it is challenging to handle the competing priorities of different stakeholders. For example, purchasers of healthcare need different information to clinicians delivering patient care or providers engaged in service design and delivery.

Guideline committees should have balanced representation from clinicians, academics, and patients, as well as public health experts and allied health professionals where relevant. The committee should be carefully recruited and trained. Expert opinion, especially in very subspecialized guideline development, is important but care must be taken to ensure that the recommendations are not biased (Morden et al., 2014).

Specialist societies are often commissioned to support guideline development. These can provide expert knowledge and experience but may sometimes also act as advocates for particular techniques or conditions. A balanced guideline committee, with patient involvement and public health experts providing a whole-population perspective and independence from specialist opinions, is desirable. The involvement of specialist societies has many advantages in development and implementation of the guidance. The credibility, dissemination, and uptake of the guidance can be improved through the reputation and membership of the society. Specialist opinion on current best practice and innovation can refine the recommendations. However, discordance of recommendations can be difficult to avoid due to differing expert opinions. To avoid bias and ensure high-quality guidance, the methods should be transparent and in line with those by such national bodies as NICE in England.

8.8 Conflicts of interest

The Institute of Medicine Committee on Standards for Developing Trustworthy Clinical Practice Guidelines recommends that any conflict of interest (COI), where financial or non-financial interests or loyalties may cause bias in development of the guideline recommendations, should be taken into account. A degree of conflict of interest may be unavoidable if a specialist clinician has expertise in a rare area of practice or a patient representative has lived experience of an illness. The Guidelines International Network recommends that all conflicts of interest should be declared and updated regularly for each member of a guideline committee. No individual with a conflict of interest should decide on the direction or strength of a recommendation (Schünemann et al., 2015). However, declaration of conflicts of interest and a transparent process of reporting any updating on them does not contribute to how potential biases caused by conflicts of interest should be handled or improved (Jones et al., 2012).

8.9 Discordant recommendations

The rigour and implementation of guideline recommendations can be hampered by disagreement between and within guideline-developing organizations (Alexander et al., 2016). Conflicting recommendations can occur for many reasons and often the conflict is a minor difference (for example, a difference about the age cut-off in recommendations from different guideline producers), but wider disagreements about treatment targets occur. Different guideline developers may produce contradictory recommendations due to limited evidence and different subgroup analyses where the sample size is small, or due to different views on current practice, settings, social factors, and resource constraints. Varied background experience of the panel members of a guideline committee can result in apparently inconsistent conclusions. For example, surgeons may have a different value system to public health professionals and health economists. So different health priorities (for example, population-based screening versus surgical intervention for treatment) may influence the guideline recommendations. Conflicting recommendations impede uptake of guidance. Mixed messages can lead to 'conflicting news' from media outlets and serious costs to public health when there is an apparent lack of consensus, as is the case in England with the use of statins for prevention of cardiovascular disease (Evans et al., 2016).

Several national and international initiatives aim to reduce the potential for conflicting recommendations. An established national organization (for example, NICE in England) may coordinate guideline production by specialist societies, royal colleges, and national collaborating centres. Individual groups should not be excluded from guideline development as constructive evidence appraisal and debate can drive healthcare improvement. Governmental organizations should also be open to challenge, new ideas, and innovative approaches. However, quality control of guidelines produced by independent groups should be addressed as a centralized, national function. For example, accreditation of the rigour of an organization's methods in producing guidelines can be given and renewed. NICE ran an accreditation programme that critically evaluated high-quality processes and identified trustworthy sources of guidance. The majority of main guidance producers in England have been accredited by NICE. Accreditation allows guidance developed by organizations to be recognized as using high-quality methodology. Criteria based on the AGREE II instrument (used to assess guideline quality) assess processes in guideline production, including external peer review and stakeholder engagement (Brouwers et al., 2016).

8.10 Updating guidance

Evidence and research is rapidly evolving and, as such, guidance can quickly become out of date. The life span of a systematic review is generally about five years (Shojania et al., 2007). The timeline for updates of guidance largely depends on the rate of innovation in the specialty covered by the guidance. Areas of rapid development include the treatment of human immunodeficiency virus and the use of biological therapy for autoimmune disease. Plans for updating guidance should be confirmed prior to development of the guidance and depend on the topic. Surveillance to check if a guideline needs to be updated can include a new review of the evidence, on either a one-off or rolling basis. Technology facilitates rolling reviews of literature through automated searches and algorithms to appraise evidence and signal implications. This type of organic or growing systematic review will smooth the update process and allow real-time incorporation of evidence into guidance.

Learning Health Systems (LHS) are emerging and may inform real-time guideline development and update. In a LHS, RWD is used alongside inputs from communities of patients, physicians, and researchers to inform quality improvement for each patient at the point of care, and data is collected at this point and fed back in

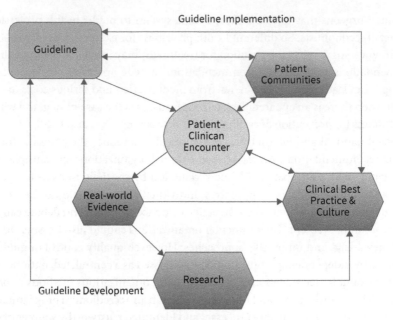

Figure 8.1 Guideline development and implementation.

to contribute to research, quality improvement, and, ideally, guideline recommendations (Forrest et al., 2014) (see Figure 8.1).

8.11 Individual patients

Individualized guidance, that addresses decisions and risk factors on an individual patient level rather than from a population perspective, is emerging. Though currently hampered by a lack of tools for risk assessment and shared decision making, advances in technology and approaches to RWD offer advances in this area.

Patient preferences should be taken into account at all points of guideline implementation, and guideline development should facilitate this process. Patient engagement in guideline development, as described here, can help incorporate patient perspectives. Inclusion of patient-reported outcomes and a focus on developing information and recommendations that are directed at individual patients can be achieved. Tools and decision aids to communicate information on the risks and benefits of interventions have been developed. (For more on patient and public involvement, see Chapter 4 in this volume.)

Shared decision making is where the patient and clinician have a two-way conversation to communicate priorities and reach a decision. Traditionally, shared decision making is used at preference-sensitive points in care; that is, where the evidence is equivocal and there is no clear weighted advantage of the benefits of intervention over the risks. In these scenarios, tools can facilitate a process where the patient and clinician discuss all evidence, recommendations, and the patient's priorities and decide together on how to proceed. The patient should feel fully informed and the clinician should facilitate the patient's exploration of personal values and preferences (Elwyn et al., 2009).

Ideally, decisions should be shared at all points in a care pathway. A precedent has been established in the courts in England following the Montgomery case, which concluded that a 'patient is autonomous and should be supported to make decisions about their own health and to take ownership of the fact that sometimes success is uncertain' (Herring et al., 2017; Royal College of Physicians and Surgeons of Glasgow, 2019). The literature on patient preference is varied and illustrates how it is important to elicit patients' preferences on an individual basis. However, there is no consensus on how to do this. Guidelines should inform patients and patient-facing material, as well as health care providers. It is recognized that clinicians need support—whether in training, tools, or information presentation—to fully identify assumptions made in the development of guidance in relation to patient preferences for particular outcomes. Guideline developers should indicate the source of recommendations and the strength of the underpinning evidence to facilitate this process. Guideline committees apply social value judgements that may differ to an individual patient's attitude to risk: for example, individuals' aversion to surgical intervention varies.

8.12 Patient involvement and engagement

In order to best accommodate individual patients' preferences, wide involvement and engagement of patients, carers, and the public is important at every stage of guideline development, from question development to implementation and evaluation planning (Montori et al., 2013). Collaboration with patients, carers, and the public can be facilitated through membership of guideline committees, testimonies, stakeholder engagement, and consultation on the scope, topic, draft, or review of guidance (NICE, 2014).

8.13 Implementing innovation

Knowledge management puts the best evidence into best practice. It aims to improve healthcare quality. Through health technology appraisal (HTA) interventions, higher efficacy and effectiveness are prioritized, and so innovation in healthcare technology, organization, and delivery is encouraged. Dissemination of guidance and knowledge supports innovation across a healthcare system and facilitates the spread of best practice. The spread of best practice and system-wide striving to implement guidance and reach established standards of care helps to reduce inequality and unwarranted variation. Evaluation of the impact of guidelines can demonstrate widespread changes in practice (Bedson et al., 2013).

8.14 Recommendations to stop or reduce interventions

While knowledge management allows innovation and supports translation of new advances in medical technology and pharmacology into daily practice, some advances in evidence find that interventions or treatments are no longer appropriate or effective. As research advances, evidence and models, theories and practices may need revision or rejection. Health technology reassessment aims to focus on managing the adoption and de-adoption of health technology throughout its life cycle. It is a mechanism that aims to improve value in healthcare through reallocation of resources from low-value to higher-value care (MacKean et al., 2013).

8.15 Guideline adaptation

In all settings, the function of guidance is to improve quality of care through establishing and applying best practice. However, the guidance must be possible to implement; it must reflect and fit with current practice and settings. The feasibility of applying guidance depends on the local context and settings. Best practice is established through guidance but, in some settings, implementation is limited by local constraints of resources, including equipment and personnel. In such cases, guideline adaptation can apply. The integrity of the evidence should be preserved as the guideline is adapted to local settings by a committee who appraise the original guideline and the local constraints. Consensus recommendations based on the original guideline but enabling implementation in the local context can be made. For example, the Indian Ministry of Health and Family Welfare supported a standardized approach to the adaptation of NICE guidance, for implementation in India (Mehndiratta et al., 2017).

8.16 Implementation

Guidelines provide a suite of systematic recommendations on best practice. Achieving the standard of healthcare set by guidelines often requires behavioural change. Implementation science is the study of methods to promote the uptake of guidance with the aim of improving quality of care. It encompasses consideration of current practice, the complexity of the setting, and the stakeholders involved in uptake of the guidance. Implementation of guidelines is challenging and can be limited in several ways. There is a delicate balance between the rigour and the ideal standards of care set by guidance, and the relevance and feasibility of implementation with individual patients and specific care settings. The function of guidance development is to improve the quality of care in a healthcare system so standards remain aspirational but also reflect and fit with current practice and setting. The reach of the guideline depends on the authors and the guideline-producing organization and their credibility amongst their intended audience (Fischer et al., 2016). Guidelines should provide advice to support decision making but, by definition, are not mandatory.

Guidelines set aspirational standards of care. Through NICE's quality standards. best practice is established and performance metrics are recommended to measure implementation and impact of the guidelines. Additionally, fundamental standards, representing the minimum baseline standard of care that healthcare providers should meet, are set by regulatory organizations and legal systems. However, guidelines are often used as standards against which the quality of care provided can be evaluated. Guidelines and quality standards inform audit programmes, where they are used to establish the benchmarks, standards, and level of quality that should be aimed for. Guidelines are also used to inform performance management and regulation of healthcare providers. Processes for implementing guidance and unjustified deviation from guidance by healthcare providers are examined, and inform regulation and licensing decisions. Healthcare providers in England are held to account by such national organizations as the Care Quality Commission, NHS Improvement, and NHS England. Clinicians are held to account by their licensing organization (for example, the General Medical Council and the Nursing and Midwifery Council) or their college or specialist society. Maintaining professional registration and a licence to practice depends on revalidation—a process in which clinicians must demonstrate how they maintain and enhance their practice by keeping up to date, as well as seek feedback from colleagues and patients. Awareness and implementation of current guidance is important for revalidation.

Though guidelines establish the optimal standards for care and aim to take into account current practice to ensure that guidance is achievable, there is still a large gap between the quality of care recommended in guidelines and the care delivered in healthcare systems every day. For example, prevention of stroke through best-practice treatment of atrial fibrillation is not universal practice (Heidbuchel et al., 2018). Many levers have been suggested and tried to address this gap. Incentives, both financial and non-financial, can be used to support guideline implementation. Best-practice awards are an example of the latter. The Quality Outcomes Framework (QOF) in England is an example of a financial incentive, where general practitioners are rewarded financially for implementing certain recommendations. It has had variable impact though (Roland & Guthrie, 2016). Vouchers for patients who breastfeed or give up smoking can be successful (Tappin et al., 2015; Johnson et al., 2018). Behavioural science techniques have been considered and tried successfully: for example, to influence prescribing practices using 'nudge' theory (Meeker et al., 2014).

Tools and resources that support the implementation of guidance can be recognized by the guideline producer as aids to better uptake of guidance. NICE runs an endorsement programme, where resources produced by external organizations can be assessed against criteria. Endorsed resources can use a NICE endorsement statement and will be published on the NICE website.

8.17 Evaluation

The implementation and impact of guidance needs to be evaluated. Guidelines contribute to evidence generation through identifying gaps in literature, describing the expected impact of interventions in the real world. The unintended consequences of interventions can be examined in careful evaluation studies of guideline impact. Guidelines can also promote the measurement of outcomes through registries and national audits.

8.18 Broader guidance—the future?

Guidelines are moving away from their traditional focus on clinical practice into new areas focusing on, for example, resource impact, systems impact, health services research, complexity, alternative treatments, and the benefits of doing nothing (Tunçalp et al., 2019). Guideline development faces many challenges: surveillance of new publications and updating, discordance amongst guideline developers, and the varied quality of final recommendations. However, developments in technology and digital architecture may begin to provide some solutions. Recommendations that can stand alone or allow patient and clinician interaction, supported by RWD and RWE to individualize risk predictions, are in development.

References

Alexander, P.E., et al. (2016). World Health Organization strong recommendations based on low-quality evidence (study quality) are frequent and often inconsistent with GRADE guidance. *J Clin Epidemiol*, 72, 98–106. doi: 10.1016/j.jclinepi.2014.10.011

Bedson, J. et al. (2013). The effectiveness of national guidance in changing analgesic prescribing in primary care from 2002 to 2009: an observational database study. *Eur J Pain*, 17(3), 434–443. doi: 10.1002/j.1532-2149.2012.00189.x

Bell, H., et al. (2016). *The use of real world data for the estimation of treatment effects in NICE decision making. Report by the National Institute for Health and Care Excellence (NICE) Decision Support Unit.* Available at: http://scharr.dept.shef.ac.uk/nicedsu/wp-content/uploads/sites/7/2017/05/RWD-DSU-REPORT-Updated-DECEMBER-2016.pdf

Brouwers, M.C., Kerkvliet, K., & Spithoff, K. (2016). The AGREE Reporting Checklist: a tool to improve reporting of clinical practice guidelines. *BMJ*, 352, i1152. doi: 10.1136/bmj.i1152

Elwyn, G., Frosch, D., & Rollnick, S. (2009). Dual equipoise shared decision making: definitions for decision and behaviour support interventions. *Implement Sci*, 4, 75. doi: 10.1186/1748-5908-4-75

Evans, S., et al. (2016). Interpretation of the evidence for the efficacy and safety of statin therapy. *Lancet*, 388(10059), 2532–2561. doi: 10.1016/s0140-6736(16)31357-5

Fischer, F., Lange, K., Klose, K., Greiner, W., & Kraemer, A. (2016). Barriers and strategies in guideline implementation–a sScoping review. *Healthcare*, 4(3), 36. doi: 10.3390/healthcare4030036

Forrest, C.B., et al. (2014). PEDSnet: a national pediatric learning health system. *J Am Med Inform Assoc*, 21(4), 602–606. doi: 10.1136/amiajnl-2014-002743

Guyatt, G.H., et al. (2008). Going from evidence to recommendations. *BMJ*, 336(7652), 1049–1051. doi: 10.1136/bmj.39493.646875.AE

Heidbuchel, H., et al. (2018). Major knowledge gaps and system barriers to guideline implementation among European physicians treating patients with atrial fibrillation: a European Society of Cardiology international educational needs assessment. *Europace*, 20(12), 1919–1928. doi: 10.1093/europace/euy039

Hernan, M.A. & Robins, J.M. (2016). Using big data to emulate a target trial when a randomized trial is not available. *Am J Epidemiol*, 183(8), 758–764. doi: 10.1093/aje/kwv254

Herring, J., Fulford, K., Dunn, M., & Handa, A. (2017). Elbow room for best practice? Montgomery, patients' values, and balanced decision-making in person-centred clinical care. *Med Law Rev*, 25(4), 582–603. doi: 10.1093/medlaw/fwx029

Hughes, L.D., McMurdo, M.E.T., & Guthrie, B. (2013). Guidelines for people not for diseases: the challenges of applying UK clinical guidelines to people with multimorbidity. *Age Ageing*, 42(1), 62–69. doi: 10.1093/ageing/afs100

Johnson, M., et al. (2018). Valuing breastfeeding: a qualitative study of women's experiences of a financial incentive scheme for breastfeeding. *BMC Pregnancy Childbirth*, 18(1), 20. doi: 10.1186/s12884-017-1651-7

Jones, D.J., et al. (2012). Conflicts of interest ethics: silencing expertise in the development of international clinical practice guidelines. *Ann Intern Med*, 156(11), 809–816, W–283. doi: 10.7326/0003-4819-156-11-201206050-00008

Kingsley, C. & Patel, S. (2017). Patient-reported outcome measures and patient-reported experience measures. *BJA Educ*, 17(4), 137–144. doi: 10.1093/bjaed/mkw060

Lawson, E.H., Gibbons, M.M., Ko, C.Y., & Shekelle, P.G. (2012). The appropriateness method has acceptable reliability and validity for assessing overuse and underuse of surgical procedures. *J Clin Epidemiol*, 65(11), 1133–1143. doi: 10.1016/j.jclinepi.2012.07.002

MacKean, G., et al. (2013). Health technology reassessment: the art of the possible. *Int J Technol Assess Health Care*, 29(4), 418–423. doi: 10.1017/S0266462313000494

Meeker, D., et al. (2014). Nudging guideline-concordant antibiotic prescribing: a randomized clinical trial toward guideline-concordant antibiotic prescribing. *JAMA Intern Med*, 174(3), 425–431. doi: 10.1001/jamainternmed.2013.14191

Mehndiratta, A., Sharma, S., Gupta, N.P., Sankar, M.J., & Cluzeau, F. (2017). Adapting clinical guidelines in India–a pragmatic approach. *BMJ (Clin Res)*, 359, j5147. doi: 10.1136/bmj.j5147

Montori, V.M., Brito, J.P., & Murad, M.H. (2013). The optimal practice of evidence-based medicine: incorporating patient preferences in practice guidelines. *JAMA*, 310(23), 2503–2504. doi: 10.1001/jama.2013.281422

Morden, N.E., Colla, C.H., Sequist, T.D., & Rosenthal, M.B. (2014). Choosing wisely–the politics and economics of labeling low-value services. *New Engl J Med*, 370(7), 589–592. doi: 10.1056/NEJMp1314965

NICE. (2014). *Developing NICE Guidelines: The Manual*. Available at: www.nice.org.uk/process/pmg20

Ogunyemi, O.I., Kim, H., Meeker, D., Ashish, N., Farzaneh, S., & Boxwale, A. (2013). Identifying appropriate reference data models for comparative effectiveness research (CER)

studies based on data from clinical information systems. *Med Care*, 51(8, Suppl 3), S45–52. doi: 10.1097/MLR.0b013e31829b1e0b

Roland, M. & Guthrie, B. (2016). Quality and Outcomes Framework: what have we learnt? *BMJ*, 354, i4060. doi: 10.1136/bmj.i4060

Rothwell, P.M. (2005). External validity of randomised controlled trials: 'to whom do the results of this trial apply?' *Lancet*, 365(9453), 82–93. doi: 10.1016/S0140-6736(04)17670-8

Royal College of Physicians and Surgeons of Glasgow. (2019). *The Montgomery Case*. Available at: https://rcpsg.ac.uk/college/influencing-healthcare/policy/consent/the-montgomery-case [accessed 29 April 2019].

Schünemann, H.J., et al. (2015). Guidelines International Network: principles for disclosure of interests and management of conflicts in guidelines. GIN principles for conflicts of interest in guidelines. *Ann Intern Med*, 163(7), 548–553. doi: 10.7326/M14-1885

Shah, K.K., Cookson, R., Culyer, A.J., & Littlejohns, P. (2013). NICE's social value judgements about equity in health and health care. *Health Econ Policy Law*, 8(2), 145–165. doi: 10.1017/S1744133112000096

Shojania, K.G., Sampson, M., Ansari, M.T., Ji, J., Doucette, S., & Moher, D. (2007). How quickly do systematic reviews go out of date? A survival analysis. *Ann Intern Med*, 147(4), 224–233.

Tappin, D., et al. (2015). Financial incentives for smoking cessation in pregnancy: randomised controlled trial. *BMJ*, 350, h134. doi: 10.1136/bmj.h134

Tunçalp, Ö., et al. (2019). Complex health interventions in complex systems: improving the process and methods for evidence-informed health decisions. *BMJ Glob Health*, 4(Suppl 1), e000963. doi: 10.1136/bmjgh-2018-000963

Vandenbroucke, J.P. (2004). When are observational studies as credible as randomised trials? *Lancet*, 363(9422), 1728–1731. doi: 10.1016/S0140-6736(04)16261-2

Wieringa, S., et al. (2018). Different knowledge, different styles of reasoning: a challenge for guideline development. *BMJ Evid Based Med*, 23(3), 87–91. doi: 10.1136/bmjebm-2017-110844

Williams, V., Boylan, A.-M., & Nunan, D. (2019). Qualitative research as evidence: expanding the paradigm for evidence-based healthcare. *BMJ Evid Based Med*, 24(5), 168–169. doi: 10.1136/bmjebm-2018-111131

World Health Organization. (2012). *Handbook for Guideline Development*. Geneva: WHO. Available at: www.who.int

9
Healthcare redesign and population health

Hugh Alderwick, Jennifer Dixon, and Jo Bibby

9.1 Introduction

Healthcare systems across the world face the challenge of redesigning services to respond to the population's changing health needs. Some of these changes are well known and widespread. Growing numbers of people are living with (and dying early from) often preventable chronic diseases. Populations are ageing, with knock-on effects for people's use of health services and the income available to pay for them. Additionally, avoidable differences in health between higher and lower socioeconomic groups persist. Yet the models of health and social care available to address these needs are often outdated, fragmented, and poorly connected to the wider social, economic, and environmental factors that play a major role in shaping health and care outcomes.

In this chapter, we describe some key considerations for healthcare redesign focused on improving population health. Healthcare is just one part of a broader system of policies, services, and conditions that influence health outcomes—from national decisions about taxation, public spending, and the allocation of resources between government programmes, to the assets in local communities that help people live healthy lives. We therefore take a systems approach—recognizing the connections between healthcare, social services, public health, and the many people and professionals interacting within them, as well as the wider factors and services that shape population health—when thinking about healthcare redesign (see Box 9.1).

The chapter is made up of four parts. The first outlines what we mean by population health and how the term has been interpreted in practice. The second illustrates why healthcare systems need to change the way they work to better address population health needs. The third outlines a broad framework for healthcare systems seeking to do this, focusing on their role in disease prevention and working with others to address the wider determinants of health. In the final section, we discuss the importance of national policy context in shaping the environment for health service redesign. Throughout, we focus on considerations for healthcare systems in high-income countries, and the examples we use are drawn primarily from the UK and USA.

Hugh Alderwick, Jennifer Dixon, and Jo Bibby, *Healthcare redesign and population health* In: *Healthcare Public Health*. Edited by: Martin Gulliford and Edmund Jessop, Oxford University Press (2020). © Oxford University Press.
DOI: 10.1093/oso/9780198837206.003.0009.

Box 9.1 Systems thinking and healthcare redesign

Systems thinking emphasizes the connections between component parts of complex systems and how they interact to produce both intended and unintended outcomes. Complex systems:

- involve multiple stakeholders (e.g. hospitals, primary care, and social services—and the staff, teams, and patients found within them);
- are adaptive to changes in their environment (e.g. clinicians changing practices in response to regulation);
- are themselves made up of and connected to other systems (e.g. hospitals are made up of multiple departments and embedded in their community).

As a result, context is crucial in understanding how complex systems work.

A systems perspective has several implications for large-scale change in healthcare (Turner et al., 2016):

- The task of redesigning services depends on coordinated action across multiple stakeholders—not just healthcare.
- Multiple mechanisms are needed at different levels to guide the process of change, such as national policy support and local management resources.
- Both the interventions and the settings they are delivered in will change over time—for example, in response to feedback on the changes implemented.

As a result, the process of change will typically span long periods of time and be fundamentally shaped by its context—not least the social context of the behaviours and cultures of the people and organizations involved.

9.2 What does population health mean?

Population health is defined as 'the health outcomes of a group of individuals, including the distribution of such outcomes within the group' (Kindig & Stoddart, 2003). Health outcomes are influenced by a wide range of factors—including socioeconomic conditions, environmental factors, individual genetics and behaviours, and access to healthcare and other services. Estimates differ, but most studies suggest that non-medical factors, like income, education, and behaviours, play a far greater role in shaping health outcomes than healthcare (McGovern et al., 2014). The distribution of health within the population is socially patterned, with those facing the harshest socioeconomic conditions consistently experiencing poorer health (Adler & Stewart, 2010).

This definition of population health has two important implications for healthcare systems. First, improving population health is not something they can do alone: addressing social, economic, and other health determinants depends on interventions at multiple levels across society. Second, improving health equity—that is, reducing avoidable differences in health within the population—is a core part of the task for health care systems seeking to improve health.

In practice, population health means different things to different people, with implications for the approach taken to improving it. For example, one study found that healthcare leaders in the USA typically used the term 'population health' to refer to the health of patients covered under health insurance contracts, while public health leaders focused on the health of whole populations in geographical areas (Noble et al., 2014). These differences are, perhaps, unsurprising, reflecting the distinct roles and incentives for healthcare and public health in the USA. So why do they matter? The risk is that a narrow interpretation of population health—with patients as the unit of analysis—may lead to approaches that focus too heavily on medical interventions for individuals, and not enough on the wider social conditions shaping health across populations.

9.3 Why do we need new service models?

While different countries face their own health challenges, healthcare systems across the globe are experiencing major changes in their population's health. The burden of disease and premature mortality has shifted from communicable diseases to non-communicable diseases (NCDs), such as heart disease and cancer. NCDs are chronic conditions that require ongoing management and support. A growing number of people live with multimorbidity—two or more chronic diseases—increasing the complexity of the support needed to keep them healthy.

The risk of chronic disease is significantly increased by unhealthy behaviours, such as tobacco use and physical inactivity—behaviours that can be modified with the right conditions and support. These behaviours, in turn, are shaped by people's social context, such as income and education, and the commercial and built environment in which they live, which act as the causes of the causes of chronic disease. One study in Scotland found that people living in the poorest areas experienced multimorbidity 10–15 years earlier than those living in the most affluent areas (Barnett et al., 2012). Populations are also ageing, with knock-on effects for their use of services: multimorbidity becomes increasingly common with age (Salisbury et al., 2011).

Broadly speaking, healthcare systems have been slow to respond to these changes. Healthcare services are largely configured to treat single diseases and episodes of care, such as hospital visits, rather than multiple NCDs requiring ongoing health and social supports. The result is that services are too often fragmented, duplicative, and imbalanced towards treating illness in hospital rather than preventing it upstream. This can lead to poor care for patients and increased costs for healthcare systems. For example, it is thought that a proportion of emergency hospital admissions (around 14% in England)—more common among patients in lower socioeconomic groups—might be avoided with better care and support in the community (Steventon et al., 2018).

At the same time, investment in services outside the healthcare sector, to address the wider determinants of health, is often lacking. Despite policy rhetoric about the importance of prevention, only around 3% of European health budgets is spent on public health (WHO Europe, 2014). Austerity policies in many countries since 2008 have made these problems worse. In England, for example, there have been cuts in spending on public health, unemployment benefits, housing, and local government services since 2010, linked to adverse health trends among some disadvantaged groups (Barr et al., 2017). Relative inequalities in mortality have generally increased in western Europe since the 1980s (Mackenbach et al., 2018).

9.3.1 Health system limits

In the face of these trends, health systems can only do so much. While greater policy attention on the role of healthcare in preventing disease is welcome, broader government decisions—for example, the level of spending on housing, working-age benefits, and other public services—will continue to influence the underlying social and economic conditions that fundamentally shape health and its distribution. Greater healthcare system involvement in addressing non-medical issues could also have unintended consequences—not least the risk of medicalizing poverty and other social issues. These risks are particularly acute in a market-based health system like that in the USA, where language and data related to patients' social circumstances could be used in ways that reduce access to care for vulnerable groups and increase inequity (Gottlieb & Alderwick, 2019).

9.4 A framework for healthcare redesign

Given these limitations, how should healthcare systems change the way they work to better address population health needs? In this section, we outline seven overlapping considerations for healthcare redesign focused on improving population health. We focus on the role of local or regional healthcare systems in preventing disease and working with other sectors to address the wider determinants of health. Given the scale and complexity of health service redesign, our approach is broad: we focus on overarching questions for healthcare leaders and policymakers (e.g. how might you think about understanding population health needs?) rather than specific interventions that could improve particular outcomes (e.g. what interventions could improve child health in context X or Y?). Our aim is to provide an overview of relevant issues and approaches, rather than a comprehensive review of the literature in each of the areas we describe.

9.4.1 Identifying population health needs

To improve population health, you first need to know where to focus. This means developing a systematic understanding of the health needs and risks within the population, including their distribution and the social and economic factors that shape them. A mix of data can be combined to do this, including on the burden of morbidity and mortality, behavioural risks, socioeconomic status and living conditions, and people's perspectives about their own health. While this kind of approach has a long history in public health, healthcare systems often focus on collecting data to identify the sickest patients or predict those at highest risk of hospital admission. Yet this kind of approach—if pursued in isolation—can miss the underlying causes of illness within the population, while underestimating the impact of service use from lower-risk groups (Rose, 2001).

A broader approach, often referred to as population segmentation, has been pursued by some health systems in Europe, the USA, and elsewhere, to better identify the varying health risks and needs within the population. For example, in 2015, the London Health Commission used data from health and social care settings, and public and staff engagement, to segment London's health needs (Vuik et al., 2016). Fifteen population groups were identified and used as a basis to plan new services, based on strengthening preventive care and better managing chronic conditions.

Advances in big data—the rapidly increasing size of available data and the speed they can be produced—are likely to offer new ways of understanding how social, behavioural, environmental, and other risks interact (and can be modified) to produce health outcomes in the future. However, smaller-scale data sharing between a handful of local agencies can also significantly increase understanding of health risks and how to address them. For example, data sharing between healthcare, police, and local government in Cardiff, Wales, has been used develop more effective violence prevention strategies in the city—including targeting police resources to violence 'hot spots' and increased frequency of late-night public transportation (Curtis et al., 2011).

9.4.2 Establishing shared objectives and measures

A related challenge to understanding population health needs is deciding how changes in health will be measured. The literature on cross-sector collaboration (see Section 9.4.6) emphasizes the importance of shared objectives and a common approach to measuring progress against them for health partnerships to operate effectively. We also know that clear goals and priorities are important for delivering high-quality care (Dixon–Woods et al., 2014). But how should this be done? In many countries, objectives for improving health already exist at a national level, set by government agencies. Yet these frameworks may only have a weak influence on local practice. Also, the measures that matter to national leaders are often skewed towards healthcare and hospitals. National health indicators may also only show a partial picture of health in any one area.

Some local health systems have developed their own objectives and measures for improving population health, designed to fit the local context. In Greater Manchester, England, where healthcare budgets have been devolved from central government, 37 health and social service organizations have agreed an overarching set of outcomes and targets for improving health and reducing inequalities by 2021. They include improving school readiness, reducing the number of low-birthweight babies and children living in poverty, reducing premature mortality, and reducing hospital admissions due to falls. Several factors need to be considered when designing local approaches to measurement, including the importance of using data with established validity and reliability, as well as some nationally available data to allow comparison. Whatever approach is taken, an explicit focus should be given to monitoring health inequalities.

Alternative approaches to measuring population health have been developed by organizations outside governments and health systems. For example, since 2010, the Robert Wood Johnson Foundation and University of Wisconsin have produced health rankings for US counties (Remington et al 2015). The rankings are based on a conceptual model of population health that includes health outcomes (e.g. life expectancy) and modifiable risk factors (covering health behaviors, clinical care, socioeconomic factors, and physical environment). Weights are applied to different domains to produce the rankings. For instance, clinical care indicators carry less weight than socioeconomic factors. Rather than being used for judgement, the aim of the rankings is to help local communities target action to improve health.

9.4.3 Aligning local resources

Historic patterns of investment and resource allocation may run against population health objectives. Resources for improving health are spread widely across sectors and communities, with healthcare services often taking a disproportionate share. Even within the health system, budgets are often fragmented—for example, between physical and mental health. This can mean that resources are not allocated efficiently to maximize health outcomes. For example, despite many public health interventions being highly cost-effective (Masters et al., 2017), they are often underfunded. On the flipside, overuse of low-value healthcare interventions is ubiquitous (Brownlee et al., 2017). A growing body of evidence also suggests that increased investment in social services, such as housing and education, is likely to have a major impact on improving population health outcomes. Several studies have found that higher ratios of spending on social services to healthcare are associated with better health (Bradley et al., 2011, 2016).

What might this mean for healthcare systems? One question is whether a greater share of healthcare resources should be invested in upstream interventions. Payment reforms in several countries have sought to change the way healthcare reimbursement works to increase incentives for providers to keep people healthy. For example, rather than being paid on a fee-for-service basis, accountable care organizations (ACOs) in the USA receive capitated budgets from health insurers to provide care for defined patient groups and to meet quality targets, including better preventive care and service coordination. Since their establishment in 2010, ACO performance has been mixed and overall quality improvements modest. However, some ACOs have developed new approaches to address patients' social needs, such as housing and food insecurity—and many have invested in care coordination for people with chronic diseases (Alderwick et al., 2018a).

Another question is whether healthcare systems could pool resources with other sectors to make a greater combined contribution to population health. Doing so has been a policy objective in several countries for decades, with varying results. Budget pooling between health and social services in England and Sweden in the 1990s and 2000s, for example, had some positive effects, including broadening managers' awareness of service interdependencies (Hultberg et al., 2005). This did not necessarily lead to changes in services, behaviours, or cultures among front-line staff though—or to improved health outcomes. Nonetheless, the benefits from more targeted regional investments could be substantial. For a mid-sized American city, modelling suggests that coordinated investments in high-quality healthcare, expanding socioeconomic opportunities, and supporting healthier behaviours could improve health, reduce inequities, and lower costs (Homer et al., 2016).

Healthcare organizations also have opportunities to use their significant economic and social capital—as employers, purchasers, and trusted institutions—to improve health and reduce inequalities in their communities. In the USA, these kinds of approaches are referred to as 'anchor institution' strategies. Examples include hospitals investing in affordable housing, early childhood development, and increased training and employment opportunities for local people.

9.4.4 Developing new service models

Even when resources are freed up for service redesign, knowing where to focus improvement efforts can be difficult. Rather than searching for 'silver bullet' solutions, health systems and policy makers are likely to have the greatest impact by focusing on reshaping the multiple components in their community that interact to influence health outcomes. For example, reducing childhood obesity requires interventions across healthcare, food, transport, education, and other systems that work together to shape calorie intake and expenditure (Rutter et al., 2017).

Within the healthcare system, various frameworks—such as the chronic care model in the USA and primary care home model in England—have been developed to help reorient care delivery towards prevention and wider services that shape health. These care models vary, but typically call for closer integration of services within the healthcare system—for example, between primary and community services, or physical and mental health—and better coordination between healthcare, social services, and wider community supports. Mechanisms proposed to do this include multidisciplinary teams, new roles such as care coordinators, and care processes like personalized care planning. Several areas in England are also pioneering new approaches to treating mental and physical ill health, such as improving physical healthcare for people with serious mental illness in primary and secondary care. In addition to new care models, ensuring equitable access to both new and existing services is equally important for tackling inequalities.

As awareness of social determinants of health has increased, a growing number of healthcare systems are experimenting with 'social prescribing' interventions. Approaches vary, but the process typically involves identifying patients' unmet social needs (e.g. food insecurity) and supporting them to access relevant non-medical services (e.g. benefits advice). While these approaches have the potential to improve health by addressing patients' social circumstances, little high-quality evidence is available on their effectiveness or to guide their implementation. Their success is also closely connected to community context. Without adequate social supports outside the health system, social prescribing risks unintended consequences—not least creating a 'road to nowhere' for vulnerable patients (Alderwick et al., 2018b).

Whatever their focus, to help new service models stick, healthcare leaders must consider the changes needed at different levels within the system that shape the context of care delivery—including at a macro (system), meso (organizational), and micro (clinical team) level. For example, encouraging clinicians to make social prescriptions (at a micro level) will be held back by limited organizational capabilities for identifying social needs (at a meso level) and conflicting accountabilities between healthcare and social services (at a macro level). At all levels within the system, a large body of evidence highlights the importance of engaging frontline staff in leading change efforts for them to have a chance of succeeding (Best et al., 2012).

9.4.5 Testing and learning

Evidence also tells us that successful service redesign requires a commitment to testing and learning (Best et al., 2012) and a systematic approach to change (Braithwaite, 2018). Because health interventions operate in a complex system, they are highly context-specific, dynamic, and social. In other words, their implementation is messy and unpredictable. As a result, ongoing cycles of testing and revision are needed to understand how services can be improved.

In practical terms, this means developing 'feedback loops' where data on the impact of interventions is shared with those designing and delivering them. This is easier said than done. If measures are too burdensome to collect or lack credibility among staff, the process risks alienating teams and creating confusion about the intervention's impact (Dixon–Woods et al., 2012). If measures become a blunt instrument for performance management rather than a tool for improvement, they risk creating perverse incentives (Bevan & Hood, 2006). Also, if measures fail to align with the wider health objectives of the system, individual interventions risk becoming fragmented and conflicting, rather than combining to direct the system towards desired outcomes. Several mechanisms are likely to support successful use of measures for health system improvement, including participation of all relevant stakeholders in defining measures, ensuring validity and trust in the data, and incentives for teams to act on their feedback (Best et al., 2012).

9.4.6 Working across systems

A key theme running throughout this chapter is the importance of healthcare systems looking beyond their own walls to consider how they can work with other sectors to improve health. The rationale for this is not hard to find. As we have described, population health outcomes are influenced by a wide range of factors, influenced by the activities of multiple organizations and groups. Cross-sector partnerships have therefore been proposed as a way to coordinate activities to improve health and health equity, and have been developed in diverse contexts.

Multiple studies have identified potential characteristics of effective cross-sector partnerships, such as shared objectives, effective communication, trust between partners, and a mix of vertical linking within sectors and horizontal linking between them (Winters et al., 2016). Despite this, evidence that these partnerships actually achieve their stated objectives—improvements in health and equity—is hard to find (Ndumbe-Eyoh & Moffat, 2013; Hayes et al., 2012). Many partnerships end up being costly, hard to manage, and struggling to navigate the cultural, organizational, and accountability issues they face. These evidence gaps can, in part, be explained by the methodological challenges of evaluating such partnerships—for example, given that they operate alongside many other policies that affect health. The result, however, is that our knowledge of how organizations can best work together to improve health is relatively limited.

9.4.7 Involving patients and communities

Finally, involving patients and communities is widely seen as an essential component for service redesign. Despite this, examples of weak patient and public involvement in healthcare are often easier to find than successful ones, and evidence that involvement leads to improvements in health outcomes is sparse (Mockford et al., 2011; Conklin et al., 2015). Nonetheless, involving the public in decisions about health services arguably has intrinsic value, and may help direct resources towards services that are most valued by people who use and pay for them.

Involvement can take place at multiple levels—from involving patients in decisions about their own care, to public involvement in health or social policy decisions. At a service delivery level, involving patients in quality improvement projects has the potential to identify gaps in services for marginalized groups, increase clinicians' understanding of how social context shapes service use, and improve service coordination. At a broader community level, involvement in decisions about health-system planning has taken various forms in the UK, USA, and elsewhere—including regional health councils, citizens' juries, and public consultations. Public deliberation approaches are increasingly being used to capture in-depth views on complex health problems (Carman et al., 2015). Deliberation may also help shift health system priorities further upstream—for example, towards community-level interventions and activities to influence social policy (Gold et al., 2018).

9.5 Conclusion

Healthcare systems across the globe have struggled to keep pace with the population's changing health needs. The growth of multimorbidity, persistent and widening health inequalities, and our increased understanding of the impact of social determinants of health all require new responses from healthcare systems and policy makers. In this chapter, we have described some of the ways that healthcare systems can think differently about their role in improving population health.

While we have focused on local or regional approaches to healthcare redesign, an important factor shaping these efforts is the national policy context in which these systems operate. National healthcare reform is governed by varying institutional logics—from 'big bang' to more incremental approaches—with implications for the direction and pace of change within them (Tuohy, 1999). Healthcare systems are also influenced by the wider choices of governments, like the level and distribution of spending on welfare benefits, housing, and other social services. A good example is the UK government's strategy to tackle health inequalities between 1997 and 2010. The strategy focused on reducing gaps in life expectancy between the poorest parts of the country and the rest. A wide range of policies were introduced to help do this—spanning better support for families, engaging communities, improving NHS prevention and treatment, and addressing social determinants of health through wider social and economic policy—combined with increased investment in the NHS, social care, and other public services, alongside broader economic regeneration strategies. Recent analysis suggests that these policies were associated with a decline in regional health inequalities, reversing a previously increasing trend (Barr et al., 2017). Fast forward a decade, however, and major cuts to local government, public health, and other social services since 2010 have held back local efforts to prioritize prevention—and may even be contributing to a reverse of the inequality reductions experienced between 1997 and 2010.

So, to put it simply, national policy matters, and changes to national health policy—to funding levels, regulation, payment systems, and more—could help guide local health systems towards more upstream approaches to improving health. However, in the meantime, clinical teams, healthcare leaders, and the communities they serve cannot afford to wait. Change within complex systems ultimately relies on the actions and interactions of the many people working within them. Individuals at all levels within the healthcare system therefore have a fundamental role to play in reshaping the way their system works—not least how it works with others in their community (such as local government, schools, and businesses)—to focus on achieving better population health, not just better healthcare. This is likely to depend as much on changes in cultures and attitudes within the healthcare system as it is on technical policy fixes.

References

Adler, N.E. & Stewart, J. (2010). Health disparities across the lifespan: meaning, methods, and mechanisms. *Ann N Y Acad Sci*, 1186, 5–23.

Alderwick, H., Shortell, S., Briggs, A., & Fisher, E. (2018a). Can accountable care organisations really improve the English NHS? Lessons from the United States. *BMJ*, 360, k921.

Alderwick, H., Gottlieb, L.M., Fichtenberg, C.M., & Alder, N.E. (2018b). Social prescribing in the U.S. and England: emerging interventions to address patients' social needs. *Am J Prev Med*, 54(5), 715–718.

Barnett, K., Mercer, S.W., Norbury, M., Watt, G., Wyke, S., & Guthrie, B (2012). Epidemiology of multimorbidity and implications for health care, research, medical education: a cross-sectional study. *Lancet*, 380(9836), 37–43.

Barr, B., Higgerson, J., & Whitehead, M. (2017). Investigating the impact of the English health inequalities strategy: time trend analysis. *BMJ*, 358, j3310.

Best, A., Greenhalgh, T., Lewis, S., Saul, J.E., Carroll, S., & Bitz, J. (2012). Large-system transformation in health care: a realist review. Milbank Q, 90(3), 421–56.

Bevan, G. & Hood, C. (2006). Have targets improved performance in the English NHS? *BMJ*, 332, 419.

Bradley, E.H., Elkins, B.R., Herrin, J., & Elbel, B. (2011). Health and social services expenditures: associations with health outcomes. *BMJ Qual Saf*, 20(10), 826–831. doi:10.1136/bmjqs.2010.048363

Bradley, E.H., et al. (2016). Variation in health outcomes: the role of spending on social services, public health, and health care, 2000–09. *Health Aff*, 35(5), 760–768.

Braithwaite, J. (2018). Changing how we think about healthcare improvement. *BMJ*, 261, k2014.

Brownlee, S., et al. (2017). Evidence for overuse of medical services around the world. *Lancet*, 390(10090), 156–168.

Carman, K.L., et al. (2015). Effectiveness of public deliberation methods for gathering input on issues in health care: results from a randomized trial. *Soc Sci Med*, 133, 11–20.

Conklin, A., Morris, Z., & Nolte, E. (2015). What is the evidence base for public involvement in health care policy? Results of a systematic scoping review. *Health Expect*, 18(2), 153–165.

Curtis, F., Shepherd, J., Brennan, I., & Simon, T. (2011). Effectiveness of anonymised information sharing and use in health service, police, and local government partnership for preventing violence related injury: experimental study and time series analysis. *BMJ*, 342, d3313.

Dixon-Woods, M., McNicol, S., & Martin, G. (2012). Ten challenges in improving quality in healthcare: lessons from the Health Foundation's programme evaluations and relevant literature. *BMJ Qual Saf*, 21(10), 876–884.

Dixon–Woods, M., et al. (2014). Culture and behaviour in the English National Health Service: overview of lessons from a large multimethod study. *BMJ Qual Saf*, 23(2), 106–115.

Gold, M.R., Realmuto, L., Scherer, M., Kamler, A., & Weiss, L. (2018). Community priorities for hospital-based prevention initiatives: results from a deliberating public. *J Public Health Manag Pract*, 24(4), 318–325.

Gottlieb, L.M. & Alderwick, H. (2019). Integrating social and medical care: could it worsen health and increase inequity? *Ann Fam Med*, 17(1), 77–81.

Hayes, S.L., Mann, M.K., Morgan, F.M., Kelly, M.J., & Weightman, A.L. (2012). Collaboration between local health and local government agencies for health improvement. *Cochrane Database Syst Rev*, 10, CD007825.

Hultberg, E.L., Glendinning, C., Allebeck, P., & Lönnroth, K. (2005). Using pooled budgets to integrate health and welfare services: a comparison of experiments in England and Sweden. *Health Soc Care Community*, 13(6), 531–541.

Homer, J., Milstein, B., Hirsch, G.B., & Fisher, E.S. (2016). Combined regional investments could substantially enhance health system performance and be financially affordable. *Health Aff*, 35(8), 1435–1443.

Kindig, D. & Stoddart, G. (2003). What is population health? *Am J Public Health*, 93, 380–383.

Mackenbach, J.P., et al. (2018). Trends in health inequalities in 27 European countries. *Proc Natl Acad Sci USA*, 115(25), 6440–6445.

Masters, R., Anwar, E., Collins, B., Cookson, R., & Capewell, S. (2017). Return on investment of public health interventions: a systematic review. *J Epidemiol Community Health*, 71(8), 827–834.

McGovern, L., Miller, G., & Hughes–Cromwick, P. (2014). Health policy brief: the relative contribution of multiple determinants to health outcomes. *Health Aff*. 10.1377/hpb20140821.404487

Mockford, C., Staniszewska, S., Griffiths, F., & Herron–Marx, S. (2011). The impact of patient and public involvement on UK NHS health care: a systematic review. *Int J Qual Health Care*, 25(1), 28–38.

Ndumbe–Eyoh, S. & Moffat, H. (2013). Intersectoral action for health equity: a systematic review. *BMC Public Health*, 13, 1056.

Noble, D.J., Greenhalgh, T., & Casalino, L. (2014). Improving population health one person at a time? Accountable care organizations: perceptions of population health—a qualitative study. *BMJ Open*, 4, e004665.

Remington, P.L., Catlin, B.B., & Gennuso, K.P. (2015). The county health rankings: rationale and methods. *Popul Health Metr*, 13, 11.

Rutter, H., et al. (2017). The need for a complex systems model of evidence for public health. *Lancet*, 390(10112), 2602–2604.

Rose, G. (2001). Sick individuals and sick populations. *Int J Epidemiol*, 30(3), 427–432.

Salisbury, C., Johnson, L., Purdy, S., Valderas, J.M., & Montgomery, A.A. (2011). Epidemiology and impact of multimorbidity in primary care: a retrospective cohort study. *Br J Gen Pract*, 61(582), e12–21.

Steventon, A., Deeny, S., Friebel, R., Gardner, T., & Thorlby, R. (2018). *Briefing: Emergency Hospital Admissions in England: Which May Be Avoidable and How?* London: The Health Foundation.

Tuohy, C.H. (1999). *Accidental Logics: The Dynamics of Change in the Health Care Arena in the United States, Britain and Canada*. New York: Oxford University Press.

Turner, S., Goulding, L., Denis, J-L., McDonald, R., & Fulop, N.J. (2016). Major system change: a management and organizational research perspective. In: R. Raine, et al. (eds) Challenges, solutions and future directions in the evaluation of service innovations in health care and public health. *Health Serv Deliv Res*, 4(16), Essay 6.

Vuik, S.I., Mayer, E.K., & Darzi, A. (2016). Patient segmentation analysis offers significant benefits for integrated care and support. *Health Aff*, 35(5), 769–775.

Winters, S., Magalhaes, L., Kinsella, E.A., & Kothari, A. (2016). Cross-sector provision in health and social care: an umbrella review. *Int J Integr Care*, 16(1), 1–19.

WHO Europe. (2014). *The Case for Investing in Public Health*. Copenhagen: WHO.

10

Programme budgeting and marginal analysis, and developing a business case for a new service

Eira Winrow and Rhiannon Tudor Edwards

10.1 Introduction: health economics

Health economics involves the use of economic theory and technique in analysing the decisions taken by all stakeholders in the production and consumption of health and social care services, be they the service users, healthcare providers, commissioners, or governments (Morris et al., 2012). It has become a specialist branch of economics based in traditional economic theory which analyses scarcity and choice, but with a theoretical body aimed specifically at understanding the behaviour of the health and social care system and of resource-allocation decision making.

As in any economic field, health economics asks three basic questions:

- What goods and services to produce?
- How to produce those goods and services?
- How to distribute goods and services between members of society?

This translates into the following three questions in a health and social care context:

- What health and social care services to produce?
- How to finance and organize the provision of these health and social care services?
- How to distribute access to health and social care amongst the population?

The demand for healthcare is infinite. As the population lives longer and technology advances, resources become scarce and choices must be made to allocate those resources efficiently. In order to prioritize services in health and social care, costs and benefits of services must be compared in order to justify those priorities and offer the best value to the public purse.

Goals of efficiency are not the only considerations for real-world decision makers in health and social care, and that is why programme budgeting and marginal analysis

Eira Winrow and Rhiannon Tudor Edwards, *Programme budgeting and marginal analysis, and developing a business case for a new service* In: *Healthcare Public Health*. Edited by: Martin Gulliford and Edmund Jessop, Oxford University Press (2020). © Oxford University Press. DOI: 10.1093/oso/9780198837206.003.0010.

(PBMA) was developed to allow decision makers to weigh up options in terms of a range of goals such as cost effectiveness, equity considerations, government priorities, public and political pressures, and the media.

10.2 The principles of programme budgeting and marginal analysis

PBMA was initially developed by the Rand Corporation in the USA in the 1950s, and was used by the American Department of Defense in the 1960s in the evaluation of military budgets and expenditure (Brambleby & Fordham, 2003). PBMA is a method that helps decision makers ensure that healthcare resources for the health needs of a local population are being maximized. The method could equally be used in social care.

Programme budgeting is an evaluation of past resource allocation within or across programmes. This allows the decision makers to review specific programmes and take decisions over whether or not those programmes should continue to be funded. Marginal analysis is the evaluation of the added benefits and costs of a suggested programme investment, or in a disinvestment context, the budget that can be released and the inevitable foregoing of benefits which results from withdrawing a healthcare programme.

Brambleby and Fordham (2003) suggest eight stages of PBMA:

1. Choose a set of meaningful programmes or initiatives.
2. Identify current activity and expenditure in those programmes/initiatives.
3. Think of improvements.
4. Weigh up incremental costs and benefits, and prioritize a list.
5. Consult widely.
6. Decide on changes.
7. Effect the changes.
8. Evaluate the progress.

PBMA may be underutilized, but we have used PBMA to improve resource allocation in the National Health Service in Wales. Box 10.1 provides an example of PBMA applied to the specialty of respiratory care. This exercise demonstrated the potential for health boards to use evidence-based approaches to reach potentially controversial disinvestment and investment decisions. The PBMA process led to disinvestment from ineffective mucolytic prescribing, while options for possible redirection of funds were explored. Box 10.2 provides an example of PBMA applied to resource allocation across the life course and across health conditions. Here, PBMA provided a transparent evidence-based tool to reach decisions about potential for disinvestment and reinvestment in health improvement strategies. It also demonstrated the potential

---

Box 10.1 Use of programme budgeting and marginal analysis (PBMA) as a framework for resource reallocation in respiratory care in North Wales, UK

Background: Since the global financial crisis, UK National Health Service (NHS) spending has reduced considerably. Respiratory care is a large cost driver for Betsi Cadwaladr University Health Board, the largest health board in Wales. Under the remit of 'prudent healthcare', championed by the Welsh Health Minister, a PBMA of the North Wales respiratory care pathway was conducted.

Methods: A PBMA panel of directors of medicines management, therapies finance, planning, public health, and healthcare professionals used electronic voting to establish criteria for decision making and to vote on candidate interventions in which to disinvest and invest.

Results: A sum of £86.9 million was spent on respiratory care in 2012–2013. Following extensive discussion of 13 proposed candidate interventions, facilitated by a chairperson, four candidates received recommendations to disinvest, seven to invest, and two to maintain current activity. Marginal analysis prioritized mucolytics and high antibiotic prescribing as areas for disinvestment, and medicines waste management and pulmonary rehabilitation for investment.

Source: data from Charles, J.M., et al. (2016). 'Use of programme budgeting and marginal analysis as a framework for resource reallocation in respiratory care in North Wales, UK'. *Journal of Public Health*, Vol. 38, Issue 3, pp. e352–e361. Oxford University Press.

---

wider application at a national level across government public health functions, to ensure resources are most cost effectively deployed, with due consideration for equity. There are several other published examples where PBMA has been applied in a national or international healthcare setting (Otim et al., 2016; Mitton & Donaldson, 2003; Twaddle & Walker, 1995).

Success in the conduct of PBMA has been defined as any of the following: participants gaining a better understanding of the area under interest; implementation of all or some of the advisory panel's recommendations; and disinvesting or resource allocation, or adopting the framework for future use (Edwards & McIntosh, 2019; Tsourapas & Frew, 2011).

Conducting a PBMA is a substantial undertaking. Identifying current spend on a 'programme' is often the greatest challenge to wider use of PBMA. Typically, programmes of interest to health services are based around disease categories (for example, 'asthma' or 'cardiovascular disease'). However, financial accounting systems do not match this concept of a programme. A hospital will typically allocate budgets, and account for spend, in departments such as radiology, outpatients, intensive care, ward

Box 10.2 A national programme budgeting and marginal analysis (PBMA) of health improvement spending across Wales: disinvestment and reinvestment across the life course

Background: Wales faces serious public health challenges, with relatively low life expectancies and wide inequalities in life expectancy, with the associated pressure on the NHS of financial recession. This has led to growing recognition of the need to better understand the range of health improvement and prevention programmes across the NHS, Welsh Government, local government, and voluntary sector agencies.

Methods: The Minister for Health and Social Care commissioned Public Health Wales (the single national public health organization) to establish a Health Improvement Advisory Group, to oversee a PBMA expert panel. The panel drew on evidence from a range of sources to explore potential alternative modes of health improvement initiative delivery across Wales. Electronic voting was used to agree an appropriate time scale for health improvement programme outcomes, the main objective of the health improvement review, and criteria for evaluating candidate services for disinvestment and investment. The panel also used electronic voting to state whether they wished to disinvest or invest in a candidate service.

Results: The review identified a budget of £15.1 million, spanning ten Welsh Government priority areas, and six life-course stages. Twenty-five initiatives were identified. The panel recommended total disinvestment in seven of these because they were not well supported by evidence; this released £1.5 million of resources. Partial disinvestment was recommended in a further three interventions, releasing £7.3 million of resources. The panel did not recommend increasing investment in any of the 25 initiatives under review. Marginal analyses prioritized child health, mental health and well-being, and tobacco control as key areas for investment.

Source: data from Edwards, R.T., et al., (2014). 'A national programme budgeting and marginal analysis (PBMA) of health improvement spending across Wales: disinvestment and reinvestment across the life course.' *BMC Public Health*, Vol. 14, Issue 1, p. 837. Springer Nature.

stays, and so on. Tracking the use of such departments and facilities by patients with a specific condition, such as asthma, is extremely difficult except in systems which use item-of-service billing, which is more usual in the private sector. Costing programmes which span primary and secondary care is also very difficult. As a result, PBMA tends to be more often used only for special projects with research input, rather than as a daily tool of healthcare public health.

10.3 How health economics is used in decision making

Health economics is much broader than merely demonstrating the efficiency or cost effectiveness of certain drugs or other health and social care interventions. Health economics can demonstrate the outcomes for a wide range of goals across many different types of programmes in many different real-world settings. The World Health Organization (WHO) uses health economics at national and international levels to provide information on effectiveness, strategic planning, policy decision making, and budget allocation, with the goal of improving health at the centre. WHO (2019) provides assistive tools such as the OneHealth online tool to enable planners in low- and middle-income countries to set specific objectives and create appropriate targets using the information they have at hand. This framework uses evidence of cost effectiveness and is hence a potentially powerful use of health economics, which allows local- and national-level decisions to be informed by real-world data.

10.4 Real-world challenges for healthcare commissioners

Health economists have not traditionally placed a focus on system change or intervention design; instead, they have focused on health technology assessment (HTA) of individual interventions or drugs. Organizations and healthcare commissioners need to build a rationale or business case for system change, and that somehow needs to include economic information about affordability and value for money, and particularly in public health, there is a pressure to demonstrate real savings. Health and social care commissioners need to build a broader case than the traditional health economics methods would allow. Therefore, health economists are more frequently engaged with decision makers to ensure that the economic considerations (evidence of cost effectiveness and equity impacts of a particular programme) are still a focus but are just one component of a real-world business case.

10.5 Building a business case for change

A business case is a document that supports proposals for a new service development or a capital project (Galloway, 2004). Making a business case for a new service, or the development or restructuring of an existing service, is an opportunity to produce a detailed written proposal for the provision of funds. A business case must clearly present all the evidence required for informed decision making, as well as providing a link between clinical and public health objectives and financial planning cycles (Galloway, 2004). At the outset, it is important that the proposal should have clear aims and objectives. Many organizations encourage the use of specific, measurable, achievable, relevant, and time-bound (SMART) objectives. This ensures that the intended targets of the development, and the extent to which they are achieved, are clear to all stakeholders.

Initially, an outline business case will be developed and, if this is accepted, then a full business case will be required. This must be informative and robust enough to be scrutinized by a decision-making body or by key decision makers, local authorities, clinical commissioning groups (CCGs), and members of the public. A business case typically compares several different options, with 'business as usual' or 'do nothing' as a comparator. An initial long list of potential ideas might be included at the outline stage and then refined to a short list of options for more detailed evaluation in the full business case.

10.5.1 Key elements of a business case

The Five-Case Model (FCM) is the method for developing business cases recommended by the UK's Treasury (HM Treasury, 2018a), the Welsh Government, and the UK's Office of Government. This model has been used widely over the last ten years, and is outlined in the UK's Treasury *Green Book* (HM Treasury, 2018b), which provides central government guidance for appraisal and evaluation of new and existing programmes. The *Green Book* suggests that business cases should be presented according to a model which views proposals from five interdependent dimensions:

- Strategic
- Economic
- Commercial
- Financial
- Management

The strategic dimension should present the rationale and objectives of the proposal, and define the current service or intervention in a 'business as usual' (BAU) scenario. These should be presented within the setting of national and local priorities and objectives, which form the strategic context for the work (Galloway, 2004).

Existing policies, government objectives, and public sector objectives should be considered at this stage. Public health input may include population health needs assessment, drawing on the local epidemiological context and comparative data, as well as evaluation of existing services, including activity levels, costs, and outcomes. Research to support the new service development presented in the strategic dimension should utilize the highest available level of evidence from evaluations of similar programmes, drawing on academic or grey literature, and recognizing gaps in existing evidence. This is where health economists can contribute evidence of cost effectiveness of new or existing programmes or services. Stakeholder engagement and public involvement undertaken at an early stage can provide understanding and insight into the current situation consistent with the 'corporate' component of a health needs assessment.

The economic dimension takes into account the value (most likely social value) of differing scenarios to the country as a whole, or the impact on a defined set of stakeholders or perspectives. The preferred choice is reached by appraisal of the different options in this economic dimension and seeks to be that which has an optimum balance of cost, benefit, and risk to society and the public sector.

The commercial dimension assesses procurement and commercial options required to implement a proposed programme, as identified in the strategic and economic dimensions.

The financial dimension discusses the net cost to the public sector at the adoption stage of a proposal, and considers all financial costs and benefits. Where the economic dimension presents social value, the financial dimension presents the financial impact on the public purse.

The management dimension presents the planning and practical arrangements for implementation and successful delivery. This dimension discusses management of the programme and resources required, and which organization would be responsible for delivering the programme. Management tools such as milestones, risk registers, and responsibility registers will also be included in this section.

10.5.2   Example of a business case

In 2010, NHS Greater Glasgow and Clyde (NHSGG&C) published an outline business case for the modernization and redesign of primary health care and community health care services (NHSGG&C, 2010). Using the Five-Case Model (with the addition of the preferred option being reported separately), NHSGG&C clearly outlined the need in that district for improved services. Box 10.3 provides a summary of the document's main conclusions as an example of the practical use of the business case process.

Box 10.3 Outline business case (OBC) for NHS Greater Glasgow & Clyde's project, 'The modernisation and redesign of primary and community health services for Possilpark'

North Glasgow experiences great poverty and deprivation, with nearly 60% of the population living in the most deprived areas in Scotland. A project was developed aiming to change the way in which healthcare was delivered to the people of the Possilpark area. Objectives included shaping health services around the needs of patients and clients through the development of partnerships between patients, carers and families, and NHS staff; and linking with local health and social care services, and with voluntary organizations and other providers, to ensure a patient-centred service. An outline business case was completed in August 2010:

Strategic case: This included a health needs assessment for the local area, linked to an overview of relevant strategic national policy documents, leading to the specification of nine SMART investment objectives.

Economic case: This developed detailed costings for each of the shortlisted options for service improvement and was accompanied by assessment of the potential benefits and risks, leading to an assessment of value for money.

Preferred option: The preferred option was the construction of a new health centre for the delivery of health services to the area. The outline business case analysed key benefits as well as service delivery considerations including service continuity, human resources, change management implications, commissioning, design, and clinical delivery.

Sustainability case: The project team analysed the sustainability of the development. The project aimed to complete a building that was designed and constructed with sustainability as a key priority, with ongoing management to continue this.

Commercial case: This addressed contractual arrangements, implementation schedules, and accountancy and charging issues.

Financial case: This examined the funding model, impact on the balance sheet, income and expenditure, and overall affordability.

Management case: This considered project management, procurement, risk management, project evaluation, and the timetable for the project.

Outcome: Construction of the new Possilpark Health and Care Centre began in November 2012, and the new centre was opened in February 2014. The development cost £10 million. The new centre incorporated four general practices, physiotherapy, podiatry, community dental services, district nursing, health visitors, social work, and health improvement teams offering smoking cessation support and sexual health services.

Source: data from 'The modernisation and redesign of primary and community health services for Possilpark'. Available at: https://www.nhsggc.org.uk/media/213771/nhsggc_obc_possilpark_2010-08-30.pdf

References

Brambleby, P. & Fordham, R. (2003). *What is PBMA? Volume 4, No. 2.* Hayward Medical Communications. Available at: http://www.bandolier.org.uk/painres/download/whatis/pbma.pdf

Charles, J.M., et al. (2016). Use of programme budgeting and marginal analysis as a framework for resource reallocation in respiratory care in North Wales, UK. *J Public Health*, 38(3), e352–e361.

Edwards, R.T. & McIntosh, E. (eds) (2019). *Applied Health Economics for Public Health Practice and Research.* Oxford: Oxford University Press.

Edwards, R.T., et al. (2014). A national programme budgeting and marginal analysis (PBMA) of health improvement spending across Wales: disinvestment and reinvestment across the life course. *BMC Public Health*, 14(1), 837.

Galloway, M.J. (2004). Best practice guideline: writing a business case for service development in pathology. *J Clin Pathol*, 57, 337–343. doi: 10.1136/jcp.2003.012518

HM Treasury. (2018a). *Guide to Developing the Programme Business Case.* London: HM Treasury. Available at: https://assets.publishing.service.gov.uk/government/uploads/system/uploads/attachment_data/file/749085/Programme_Business_Case_2018.pdf

HM Treasury. (2018b). *The Green Book: Central Government Guidance on Appraisal and Evaluation.* London: HM Treasury. Available at: www.gov.uk/government/uploads/system/uploads/attachment_data/file/220541/green_book_complete.pdf

Mitton, C.R. & Donaldson, C. (2003). Setting priorities and allocating resources in health regions: lessons from a project evaluating program budgeting and marginal analysis (PBMA). *Health Policy*, 64(3), 335–348.

Morris, S., Devlin, N., & Parkin, D. (2012). *Economic Analysis in Health Care.* John Wiley.

NHS Greater Glasgow and Clyde. (2010). Modernisation and redesign of primary and community health services for Possilpark. Available at: https://www.nhsggc.org.uk/media/213771/nhsggc_obc_possilpark_2010-08-30.pdf

Otim, M.E., Asante, A.D., Kelaher, M., Anderson, I.P., & Jan, S. (2016). Acceptability of programme budgeting and marginal analysis as a tool for routine priority setting in Indigenous health. *Int J Health Plan Manag*, 31(3), 277–295.

Tsourapas, A. & Frew, E. (2011). Evaluating 'success' in programme budgeting and marginal analysis: a literature review. *J Health Serv Res Policy*, 16(3), 177–183.

Twaddle, S. & Walker, A. (1995). Programme budgeting and marginal analysis: application within programmes to assist purchasing in Greater Glasgow Health Board. *Health Policy*, 33(2), 91–105.

World Health Organization (WHO). (2019). *Cost Effectiveness and Strategic Planning (WHO-CHOICE).* Available at: https://www.who.int/choice/onehealthtool/en/

11
Evaluating healthcare systems and services

Edmund Jessop

11.1 Introduction: dimensions for evaluation

A doctor may wonder 'Am I a good doctor? Do I serve my patients well?', but in public health we ask 'Is this a good healthcare system? How well does it serve its population?' There are many ways to answer these questions, but we can start with the idea that a healthcare system should save life and relieve suffering, and treat people with care, dignity, and respect, while doing no harm. Within each of these three areas, there are many aspects to explore. Saving life includes the immediate drama of stopping a torrential haemorrhage, but also includes the less obvious and longer-term objective of preventing cardiovascular disease by treating high cholesterol levels. Relief of suffering includes prompt and adequate analgesia for acute pain, but also includes a much wider discourse about quality of life. Care and dignity encompass kindness, the giving of information, responsiveness to questions, acceptable wait times, hospital food, and much else. These main domains are recognized in the UK's NHS Outcomes Framework, which was established through public consultation and includes the objectives of preventing people from dying prematurely, enhancing the quality of life for people with long-term conditions, helping people to recover from episodes of ill health or following injury, ensuring that people have a positive experience of care, and treating and caring for people in a safe environment and protecting them from harm.

Within these main domains of healthcare outcomes, where should we direct our attention and which aspects of healthcare should we evaluate? This is not a new question: 50 years ago, Klein (1961) interviewed health officials and identified a list of 80 evaluation criteria. Twenty years later, Maxwell (1984) considered that there were six key dimensions, as shown in Box 11.1. Maxwell's list is strongly influenced by public health thinking. Effectiveness and social acceptability matter for the individual patient, but the dimensions of access, fairness, and relevance to community needs set healthcare in a population context. We may ask whether it is right to include efficiency or value for money as measures of healthcare quality, but any government or healthcare payer will need to know whether the resources allocated to the healthcare system are justified in terms of the opportunity costs represented by alternative potential uses of resources. Maxwell's thinking was grounded in the perspective of the UK National

Edmund Jessop, *Evaluating healthcare systems and services* In: *Healthcare Public Health*. Edited by: Martin Gulliford and Edmund Jessop, Oxford University Press (2020). © Oxford University Press. DOI: 10.1093/oso/9780198837206.003.0011.

Box 11.1 Dimensions for evaluation of health services

Dimension	Description
Effectiveness	Extent to which a healthcare intervention achieves the intended outcome (Last, 2007)
Efficiency	Outcome achieved in relation to expenditure of resources (Last, 2007)
Equity	Fairness, or justice, in respect of treatment of different individuals or groups
Access	Extent to which services are available, can be utilized and delivered, and achieve appropriate outcomes
Appropriateness	Relevance to need
Responsiveness	Social acceptability

Adapted with permission from Maxwell, R.J. 'Quality assessment in health'. *BMJ (Clin Res Ed)*. Vol. 288, pp. 1470–2. Copyright © 1984 BMJ Publishing Group Ltd

Health Service, in which healthcare is generally provided free of charge at the point of use, but in most health systems, the affordability of services will also be a key concern. Maxwell's dimensions find continuing application in health system evaluation. The American Commonwealth Fund (2011) employs a scorecard approach, with multiple indicators for the domains of 'healthy lives', 'quality of care', 'healthcare access', health system efficiency', and 'equity'.

11.2 Evaluating an existing service: Donabedian's framework

Donabedian (1966 and 2003) proposed a framework for evaluating health services based on structure, process, and outcome which is still in wide use. Donabedian described structure as 'concerned with such things as the adequacy of facilities and equipment; the qualifications of medical staff and their organization; the administrative structure and operations of programs and institutions providing care; fiscal organization and the like' (Donabedian, 1966, p. 170). Nowadays, we would expand this list to include indicators of access such as the location and opening hours of the facilities, and the qualifications of all professionals, not just the medical staff. However, we could still agree with his comment that 'this approach offers the advantage of dealing, at least in part, with fairly concrete and accessible information. It has the major limitation that the relationship between structure and process or structure and outcome, is often not well established' (Donabedian, 1966, p. 170). Structure as a measure of health services has the unique advantage that it can be measured in advance. The structural features of a service can be written into a specification or contract before the service starts: process and outcome measures are only known once the service is treating patients, which may be too late. Stretching the definition of 'structure' slightly, we could include here the written protocols for treating a patient. Of course, we still need to check that what was promised in the contract is actually delivered in terms of contract compliance.

Evaluation of process describes the activity of the service, including who is being treated and what is being done to them. This may incorporate information on numbers of patients; their age, sex, and ethnicity; their diagnoses; and their comorbidities. This enables evaluation of the demographic characteristics of the patients attending the service and whether this is consistent with the distribution of need and the known epidemiology of the disease in the local population. A deficit of young or very old patients, an imbalance of male and female, or a lack of people from ethnic minorities may indicate problems of access for particular types of patients. Evaluation of diagnostic categories can be informative. If referrals to a local neurology service are dominated not by the diseases of neurology textbooks but by headache, this can raise important questions about appropriate use of highly trained, scarce, and costly specialists.

Process information also comprises what was done to the patient, including tests, procedures, and interventions delivered. A key aim is to ensure that processes of care cover effective interventions, identified from randomized trials, that can be translated into routine clinical practice for all eligible patients. Healthcare is increasingly organized around evidence-based standards of care that can be readily audited. The Quality Outcome Framework for primary care in England has been described as the largest pay-for-performance scheme anywhere in the world (Roland, 2004). A major focus of the scheme was on ensuring that all patients with selected long-term conditions achieve evidence-based standards for processes and intermediate outcomes of care. When introduced, it focused almost entirely on what had been measured or recorded, rather than the health status of patients, although over time, greater consideration has come to be given to the latter. Increasingly, care bundles and care pathways are used as markers of good care. The 'Surviving Sepsis' campaign has described a care bundle for critically ill patients with sepsis. Kutz et al. (2018) defined a care bundle for the annual review of patients with diabetes, and used it to audit and improve care.

Donabedian's third category for evaluation is outcome—in terms of the changes in health that are attributable to healthcare intervention. Donabedian recognized outcome as the most important dimension, but this is also the most difficult dimension to evaluate. Firstly, it may be difficult to identify and measure the components of health status that are responsive to healthcare. Secondly, it will usually be difficult to attribute changes in population health status to health services rather than other determinants of health. Epidemiological study designs permit estimation of a counterfactual because data from a control group show what might have happened in the absence of the intervention. Health service evaluations often lack comparators that provide counter-factual data. In the following paragraphs, we discuss how routinely collected data may be used in health services evaluations, with a particular focus on health outcomes of healthcare.

11.3 Population mortality

The first priority for a health system is to save life. In consequence, mortality rates are a primary indicator of how well a healthcare system is performing. Information on mortality requires careful analysis and interpretation. Students of public health need no reminding that for many populations in the world, housing, food supply, and sanitation drive mortality more strongly than healthcare quality. Even when the basics of shelter, food, and water are assured, social and economic factors may be dominant influences on population mortality. However, there are some illnesses that should cause few if any deaths in the twenty-first century; something may be wrong with the health-care system of a country with very high mortality from tuberculosis, appendicitis, or diabetes because these conditions should be treatable with modern medicine and surgery. These causes of death may not be completely eradicable, or always preventable, but should seldom be fatal in the modern era. Charlton et al. (1983) proposed a list of conditions which should be 'amenable to medical intervention' and showed that there was substantial variation in avoidable mortality between geographical areas. The idea of mortality 'amenable to medical intervention' was widely adopted and later expanded to include diseases which may not be treatable but are preventable, perhaps by public health action; the combination of 'amenable' with 'preventable' forms the category of 'avoidable' deaths. In middle- and low-income countries that often lack universal health coverage, there is a high burden of amenable mortality. Analysis of data from the 2016 Global Burden of Disease Study showed that there were 8.6 million excess deaths per year amenable to healthcare, including 5.0 million from receipt of poor-quality care and 3.6 million from non-utilization of healthcare (Kruk et al., 2018).

11.4 In-hospital mortality

Although use of mortality to evaluate healthcare systems at national and regional levels is now widely accepted, using death rates to judge quality of care in individual hospitals remains controversial. The mix of patients admitted varies widely between hospitals, and available data may not be sufficient to enable satisfactory risk adjustment (Lilford & Pronovost, 2010). The NHS in England now publishes summary hospital-level mortality indicator (SHMI) reports. These employ a standard method which compares the observed number of deaths with the number expected based on the characteristics of admitted patients including age, gender, comorbidity, specialty, emergency status, and season (Campbell et al., 2012). There are several criticisms of this indicator, which characterizes each hospital in England by a single number. Firstly, it does not work well for large hospitals with many different specialties and departments; good and bad alike are aggregated together into a single indicator. Secondly, death in hospital is infrequent, so the indicator misses most of what the hospital actually does. Deaths may also be expected if the patient has been admitted for end-of-life care. The SHMI excludes the latter category, but only if coded as such in the hospital's discharge data, which makes it vulnerable to coding anomalies.

There is evidence that the SHMI is associated with the socioeconomic status of the population which the hospital serves. This might suggest that poor areas are served by poor hospitals, but it is also likely that the all-pervasive influence of deprivation on health status is an unmeasured confounder of the analysis, and so the SHMI may not be a fair measure of what goes on inside the hospital.

Some of these difficulties are reduced if, instead of a hospital-wide, all-activity indicator, analysis focuses on a single specialty or a single intervention. Even so, adjusting for case mix is a key problem. 'Case mix' may refer to the mix of different diseases or operations, or it may mean the mix of complexity and severity of patients within an apparently homogeneous category. In intensive care and trauma, severity scores have been developed to allow expected mortality (given how ill each patient was at admission) to be compared with actual mortality. In cardiac surgery, a more common approach is to restrict the analysis to a particular type of operation (e.g. valve replacement or coronary artery surgery).

11.5 Quality of life

Healthcare services should improve, or at least mitigate, the impact of illness and disease on quality of life. Knowing whether healthcare services achieve that goal is hugely difficult, both conceptually and in practice. Many authors have explored questions of what is meant by 'quality of life' and how it may be measured (Streiner et al., 2014). Most writers agree that self-reported measures are essential, even though they are by nature subjective. A wide range of patient-reported outcome measures (PROMs) have been developed for use in healthcare settings (Bowling, 2017). These are generally divided into generic and condition-specific measures, and examples are presented in Table 11.1. Generic measures have the advantage that they provide metrics that can be compared across different areas of healthcare, but may not be sufficiently detailed to evaluate the impact of a given health condition. They often focus on producing a single summary score for quality of life that can be employed in health economic evaluation; condition-specific measures are more commonly used to assess the impact of illness across multiple dimensions, with separate scores.

Development and use of health-related quality-of-life measures requires appreciation of the role of psychometric theory in evaluating the reliability and validity of measures (Streiner et al., 2014). Particular concerns include whether measures are

Table 11.1 Quality-of-life measures

	Measure	Main dimensions
Generic	Medical Outcomes Study Short Form 36 (SF36) (Ware et al., 1996)	Vitality, physical functioning, bodily pain, general health perceptions, physical role functioning, emotional role functioning, social role functioning, mental health
	EuroQol (EQ5D) (1990)	Mobility, self-care, usual activities, pain/discomfort, anxiety/depression
Condition-specific	Western Ontario and McMaster Universities Osteoarthritis Index (WOMAC) (Lundgren–Nilsson et al., 2018)	Pain, stiffness, functional limitation
	Quality-of-life measure for patients with dentofacial deformity (Orthognathic Quality-of-Life Questionnaire) (Cunningham et al., 2000)	Social aspects, facial aesthetics, function, awareness of facial deformity

responsive to changes in health over time, whether there is evidence of response shift from participants' recalibration of their responses, and whether instruments perform differently in population subgroups.

In the UK, the NHS has been continuously measuring PROMs for selected procedures since 2009. For hip and knee replacement, assessment includes both a generic measure (EQ5D) and a condition-specific measure (Oxford Score), with risk-adjusted scores being reported. The fact that this programme, although running since 2009, only covers a few procedures across the whole of healthcare shows how difficult assessment is. Key problems include loss to follow-up (patients are rarely fully recovered at the time of hospital discharge and so ascertaining the true outcome of care requires data to be collected long after discharge) and the difficulty of ensuring self-completion across a broad range of patients. Information is also published on the outcome of every consultation in the Improving Access to Psychological Therapies Programme, by using valid depression (PHQ-7) and anxiety (GAD-9) questionnaires. Remarkably, this information is recorded for 98% of the 500,000 patients treated each year in the NHS in England (Clark et al., 2018), perhaps because, unlike the surgical PROMs, it is recorded while patients are still under care, not several months later.

We are still at a very early stage of using quality-of-life measures to evaluate healthcare services. In non-randomized studies, it may be very difficult to interpret these data. What counts as good or bad? How much improvement could we realistically expect in patients' quality of life, as measured by these scores? If patients at hospital

A are scoring higher or lower than at hospital B, is that telling us about the quality of healthcare or something more global in their lives?

11.6 Patient experience

It may seem obvious that the best way to evaluate a healthcare service is to ask patients what they think, but patients may find it difficult to judge whether the technical quality of care they have received is satisfactory (Rao et al., 2006). Indeed, patients seem to look for aspects other than technical competence when judging healthcare quality. The British GP Harold Shipman was convicted of murdering 15 of his patients, but some of his patients regarded him as an excellent GP: 'I remember the time Shipman came to my Dad. He would come around at the drop of a hat. He was a marvellous GP apart from the fact that he killed my father' (Hurwitz & Vass, 2002). Patients are certainly able to judge the experience of care they receive, and patient experience data is now an important element of several healthcare systems. In the USA, the Centers for Medicare and Medicaid Services require the use of a standardized patient experience measure in hospitals that treat Medicare and Medicaid patients. The Hospital Consumer Assessment of Healthcare Providers and Systems (HCAHPS) includes 32 items (questions) concerning patients' experiences including communication with doctors and nurses, responsiveness of hospital staff, pain management, communication about medicines, discharge information, cleanliness and quietness of the hospital environment, and transition of care. This dataset now drives a small element of the reimbursement hospitals receive from Medicaid. Communication from doctors and nurses is prominent in patient experience surveys mandated by the English NHS, but HCAHPS is unusual in its attention to cleanliness and quietness.

In the English NHS, sample data from a general practice assessment questionnaire is mandatory under the general practice contract and contributes to reimbursement (Ramsay et al., 2000). This assessment focuses on access, technical care, communication, interpersonal care, trust, knowledge of the patient, nursing care, receptionists, and continuity of care (Ramsay et al., 2000). As with quality-of-life data, use of patient experience information for healthcare evaluation is limited, though within an institution or system, and over time, such information becomes actionable.

11.7 Patient safety

Hippocrates' maxim 'First, do no harm' is still relevant 2,000 years later, and evaluation of a healthcare system must pay attention to harm as well as benefit. For a long time, the harms caused by medical intervention were unacknowledged, and the criticisms of radical writers like Illich (1976) were unheeded. In the USA, large studies showed that medical errors and adverse events were much more common than previously expected, leading to an estimate that 98,000 Americans die in hospital each

---

Box 11.2 Definitions of patient safety, errors, and adverse events

---

- **Patient safety:** the prevention of errors and adverse effects to patients associated with healthcare.
- **Error:** the failure of a planned action to be completed as intended (error of execution) or the use of a wrong plan to achieve an aim (error of planning).
- **Adverse event:** an injury caused by medical management rather than the underlying condition of the patient.
- **Preventable adverse event:** adverse event attributable to error.

Source: data from Kohn, L.T. et al. (2000). 'To err is human: building a safer health system'. Washington, DC: National Academy Press. National Academy Press.

---

year as a result of medical errors (Starfield, 2000). In 2000, the American Institute of Medicine threw new light on issues of medical error and patient safety through its report entitled 'To err is human' (Kohn et al., 2000). This report was important in defining medical errors and adverse events (Box 11.2), in helping to understand why errors happen, and in showing the importance of learning from errors and adverse events in order to improve the safety of health systems. Errors are not usually the responsibility of 'bad' practitioners but of 'good' practitioners working within defective systems.

Adverse effects of medication account for a large proportion of admissions to hospitals, particularly among old people, but routine monitoring usually focuses on the more catastrophic examples of harm such as avoidable death, wrong-site operations, and mismatched blood transfusions. These have come to be known as 'never' events—events which should literally never happen. This concept was developed in the USA and later adopted elsewhere. The original list of 'never' events set out by the National Patient Safety Agency in England contained eight such events (Box 11.3). Recent developments include a longer list of 'never' events and the addition of near misses as well as actual events. The occurrence of a 'never' event should trigger two consequences—an inquiry into what happened, preferably in the form of a root-cause analysis, and a report to an external authority such as the relevant public health agency. This external reporting is important, to give accountability.

Root-cause analysis is used in many industries. An event may have an obvious cause but getting to the root of the problem—the underlying issue which triggered the sequence of events—may take systematic, detailed investigation. One technique for getting to the root cause is to ask the question 'why?' five times (Box 11.4). In the example cited in Box 11.4, what looked at first sight as incompetence on the part of the surgeon turns out to have causes rooted deeper in the system: blaming the surgeon will not prevent the same thing happening again, perhaps next time with a different service or in a different area. One practical problem with 'never' event reporting is that each event

---

Box 11.3 'Never' events identified by the UK National Patient Safety Agency

---

1. Wrong-site surgery
2. Retained instrument post operation
3. Wrong-route administration of chemotherapy
4. Misplaced nasogastric or orogastric tube not detected prior to use
5. Inpatient suicide using non-collapsible rails
6. Escape from within the secure perimeter of medium- or high-security mental health services by patients who are transferred prisoners
7. In-hospital maternal death from post-partum haemorrhage after elective Caesarean section
8. Intravenous administration of mis-selected concentrated potassium chloride

---

can seem to be the result of a unique set of circumstances coming together—hence no learning for elsewhere. 'Never' events are by definition extremely rare and it can be difficult to spot common factors, especially if they are important but nebulous—for example, poor leadership or lack of a strong safety culture in the hospital.

11.8 Indicator sets

The data produced through health systems are now being analysed to develop health indicator datasets. An effective indicator set should allow us to answer three key questions:

- Which problems are big and which are small?
- Are things getting better or are they getting worse?
- Where do we stand in relation to everyone else? (Kelly & Hurst, 2006)

Box 11.4 Example of root-cause analysis

---

1. *Why was the wrong limb amputated?* Because the surgeon made an error.
2. *Why did the surgeon make this error?* Because it wasn't obvious, clinically, which limb needed amputation.
3. *Why wasn't it obvious?* Because the correct limb wasn't marked.
4. *Why wasn't the limb marked properly?* Because the ward had run out of indelible marker pens.
5. *Why had they run out?* Because the ward clerk was on sick leave and her duties, including ordering the resupply of marker pens, had not been reassigned.

An ideal indicator set would be comprehensive, covering all relevant dimensions; universal, covering all entities in the health system; and timely, providing up-to-date information. The universal aspect of an ideal indicator set is particularly important in public health, since partial indicators that cover only a select few might exclude groups in most need. In practice, it is difficult to develop indicators which perfectly meet all requirements.

Problems of classification, coding, and comparability affect the interpretation of many indicator sets. Some of these problems are quite subtle and require detailed knowledge of the underlying data: it is a good rule to consult an individual with expert knowledge of the data before reaching firm conclusions. For example, European countries have different definitions of viability and hence different rules for classifying live birth, stillbirth, and abortion (Masuy–Stroobant & Gourbin, 1995). This affects not only perinatal and infant mortality statistics but also calculations of life expectancy, with potentially large impacts on a wide range of analyses and comparisons. Even within a single country, coding and classification problems may arise. Pemberton and Cust (1986) noted a great excess of death from osteoporosis in one area of England; the explanation was a single coroner (medical examiner) who felt that most deaths following fractured neck of femur should be attributed to osteoporosis.

Coding and classification artefacts can also skew trend data, and adjustments must be made as each new revision of the International Classification of Diseases is introduced. Even when diagnosis, coding, and classification are uniform, international comparisons require expert interpretation. Median age at death has been used as a marker of care quality in genetic disorders such as cystic fibrosis; but the prevalent mutations differ between countries, with milder forms of the disease being commoner in some jurisdictions. Comparisons of performance in solid-organ transplant are affected by the quality of donor organs: partly because of high rates of death due to firearms, donors in the USA are on average younger (and hence provide higher-quality organs) than in Europe.

In addition to problems of coding, classification, and comparison, there are also problems with the statistical behaviour of league tables. Goldstein and Spiegelhalter (1996) have discussed the mathematics of this but, in essence, the problem is that small random variations can hugely affect one's position in a ranking or league table. This is particularly unfortunate given the natural tendency of human beings to put everything in a ranking or league table.

11.9 Healthcare audit

The dictionary definition of an audit is 'a systematic review or assessment'. Audit is usually a cyclical process of setting standards and criteria, measuring the level of performance, making improvements, and determining whether these are maintained.

A general practice may decide to audit wait times for routine appointments and find that 80% of patients wait two days or less, 15% wait three to seven days, and 5% wait more than seven days. The full benefits of audit are not realized unless some action is taken to improve wait times. The practice may decide to set a standard that no patient should wait more than seven days, and so create capacity for more routine appointments. This action should be followed by another round of data collection to see if the action has solved the problem. Quality improvement activity is now a mandatory requirement for medical practitioners in the UK, in order for them to keep their licence to practice, and so audits are a routine part of medical practice in all specialties. There are also several large national audits: for example, in myocardial infarction (Bebb et al., 2017) and stroke (Bray et al., 2018). However, audits will be mostly designed and executed by teams within individual hospitals or facilities.

The audit process is most likely to produce improvement when the assessment is made against a clearly defined, numerical benchmark or standard. The benchmark may be arbitrary, evidence-based, or comparative. An arbitrary benchmark might, for example, be formulated as 'no patient is to wait more than four hours in the hospital emergency department'. Clearly. long waits are bad, but the choice of four hours for the benchmark is arbitrary. There is, however, published research on door-to-needle time in coronary revascularization, so the one-hour benchmark for this process is evidence-based. Comparative benchmarks may take the form of aiming to be in the top quartile for performance. The availability of published evidence, or of data from other hospitals, will guide the choice of comparative benchmarks; if neither are available, an arbitrary benchmark is needed. Donabedian's framework can be used to develop benchmarks for structure, process, or outcomes. For example: structure, 'the multidisciplinary team will include a named clinical psychologist'; process, 'all core members of the team will attend the weekly meeting'; outcome, 'wound infection rates will be less than 0.5%'.

Acquiring the information needed for the audit is time-consuming, and most large hospitals now have an audit team to help the clinical teams design and execute their audits. Retrospective audits are the norm, which typically require the retrieval of medical records and manual searching to find the relevant information. Electronic records should be easier to retrieve and search, but often they are not. The key problem with prospective audits is one of compliance—clinicians are always busy and may forget, or not have time, to record the audit information.

11.10 Confidential enquiries

Confidential enquiries are another way to evaluate and respond to avoidable harm in health systems, with an explicit goal of sharing experience and learning. The longest-running one is the Confidential Enquiry into Maternal Deaths, established in the UK in the 1950s. This confidential enquiry involves four steps:

1. Reporting of the maternal death to trigger the enquiry.
2. Obtaining written statements of their actions from all professionals involved in care of the mother (e.g. obstetrician, midwife, GP, social worker), with a guarantee of confidentiality.
3. Assessment of statements by external experts, who note actions and omissions which might have contributed to the death.
4. Compiling an annual report to identify common themes or areas for action nationwide.

The requirement for confidentiality is important, to allow professionals to give a full and honest account, but full confidentiality may be impossible to guarantee. In the UK, the government granted full protection from legal disclosure for the written statements from professionals for the Confidential Enquiry into Maternal Deaths (but only to this specific enquiry).

A recent report noted a number of maternal deaths from influenza and identified that pregnant women are particularly vulnerable to this infection. The report emphasized the importance of both influenza vaccination for pregnant women and prompt use of antiviral drugs including neuraminidase inhibitors (Maternal, Newborn, and Infant Clinical Outcome Review Programme, 2014). Confidential enquiries are very time-consuming to compile and analyse: they are best suited to outcomes or events which are both fairly rare and serious. The method has been used nationwide in England to evaluate perinatal death, perioperative deaths, and certain categories of suicide. More recently, it was used in a county jurisdiction (Somerset) to evaluate care of patients with learning disabilities; the report highlighted several deficiencies in the care of physical illness among such people (Heslop et al., 2013).

11.11 When to act

Sooner or later, evaluation will uncover a situation that requires action, and typically at a particular hospital or facility. Sometimes the action required is to offer congratulations or award a prize for excellence, but more often we need to take action on poor performance, with remediation, suspension, or cessation of a service. The decision to act is a high-stakes one which needs careful deliberation. A basic deliberation process might consist of five stages: confirming the facts and gathering informal information, applying a decision rule, formal investigation, issuing a report, making and implementing a decision.

Confirming the facts includes checking all of the relevant data for completeness and accuracy. If, for example, a service appears to have a high mortality rate, it is important to check the denominator as well as the numerator. A surgical service with apparently high mortality (case-fatality ratio) may have reported all of their deaths promptly (numerator) but not be to date with the apparently less urgent task of reporting their successful operations (denominator). This undercount of successful operations causes an upward bias in estimating the mortality rate. Data which triggered concern may be regarded as index data. Preliminary fact finding should include a look at whether the problem is an isolated incident or blip, or whether it is part of a wider, consistent pattern. If there is a drop in performance, does it affect all patients or only one category? Has it happened before or is this the first time? Does it affect all hospitals or just one?

It is also important to go wider than just the numbers in assessing the situation. In particular, nurses are a good source of information on quality of service. Poor performance by paediatric cardiac surgeons in Bristol was first highlighted by an anaesthetist (Dyer, 2001); an ophthalmologist seeing early and severe diabetic eye disease may comment on the diabetic service in a hospital. Sometimes the whistle is blown when a patient moves hospital and the new team are dismayed to see what their predecessors have done. Cultivating a wide range of informal contacts, so as to access this type of information, is an important part of service evaluation in the real world.

A decision rule, agreed in advance and applied across all services, can help to ensure orderly decision making. Agreeing the rule in advance, and not when the problem arises, helps to secure the cooperation of the service under investigation. A common rule is to investigate further when the performance of a unit lies outside the 95% confidence interval of the national average or other reference number.

If the decision rule confirms an actionable situation, the next step is a detailed fact-finding investigation (either internally within the service, or preferably with external assistance) of the trigger events. For example, the trigger may have been five deaths over a period. The investigation may then focus on those five deaths, perhaps using confidential enquiry methodology. Written terms of reference are helpful to limit the scope of the enquiry, though the investigation may reveal a much wider problem than was realized initially. Sometimes a retrospective look at all patients treated within the service during a specified period (and not just the index patients) may become necessary.

A written report of findings from the formal investigation is important, and it is good practice for the investigation team to be separate from the person or team which has responsibility for the action decision.

11.12 Evaluation of a new system: research

So far we have been discussing the evaluation of existing health services and systems, but we may want to evaluate a new or proposed service using research designs. In principle, all of the standard research designs are available—descriptive studies, time series, intervention studies, modelling, and so on—with their usual strengths and weaknesses. The study of healthcare systems does, however, impose some constraints. It is, for example, almost impossible to randomize patients individually to receive a completely new system of healthcare involving a whole jurisdiction. Before and after comparisons, or case-comparator studies, are more feasible; qualitative designs may also provide useful insights.

That said, evaluation is always better than no evaluation, especially since governments are prone to introduce entirely untested schemes particularly when elections loom. There is no space here for a full review of health services research, but some examples may give a flavour of what can be done, and why the results are sometimes counter-intuitive.

The RAND health insurance experiment is an example of a randomized controlled trial. This study, which ran in the USA for 15 years from 1974, is probably the largest study ever conducted of healthcare financing. About 5,000 patients were individually randomized to receive free care or to different levels of co-payment. Some years later, the lead investigator summarized his findings as follows:

> For most people enrolled in the RAND experiment, who were typical of Americans covered by employment-based insurance, the variation in use across the plans appeared to have minimal to no effects on health status. By contrast, for those who were both poor and sick—people who might be found among those covered by Medicaid or lacking insurance—the reduction in use was harmful, on average.
>
> (Newhouse, 2004, p. 108)

In the late 1980s, there was growing concern about delays in hospital emergency departments. The key problem appeared to be wait times to see a doctor, hence delaying treatment for some acutely ill patients. Some hospitals responded by appointing specialist nurses to do the initial triage of patients, reasoning that this would mean seriously ill patients could be fast-tracked to the doctors. George et al. (1992) examined this belief, using an on/off (or case-comparator) design within a single emergency department, comparing periods when the nurse triage system was operating against times when it was not (due to staffing constraints). The research team reached the counter-intuitive conclusion that introducing nurse triage 'may impose additional delay, particularly among patients needing the most urgent attention' (George et al., 1992).

Qualitative methods may also be used to research new systems of healthcare, with the advantage of finding out not just whether something works, but how and why. Greenhalgh et al. (2018) looked at telemedicine, and specifically outpatient video consultations in diabetes and cancer surgery. Telemedicine is being widely advocated as an option to improve efficiency in the hospital and promote self-efficacy for patients, who can thus avoid the burden of travel to specialist hospitals and clinics. The reality, as found by the research team, was that video consultation may be a useful option but it is not the answer to all problems:

> The reality of establishing video outpatient services in a busy and financially stretched acute hospital setting proved more complex and time-consuming than originally anticipated. By the end of this study, between 2% and 22% of consultations were being undertaken remotely by participating clinicians. In the

remainder, clinicians chose not to participate, or video consultations were considered impractical, technically unachievable, or clinically inadvisable. Technical challenges were typically minor but potentially prohibitive.

(Greenhalgh et al., 2018)

These examples show that research evaluations of healthcare systems are both possible and necessary, though I should add that in all three instances cited here, the findings were strongly contested. Good research puts a brick in the wall of knowledge but it does not settle all controversies.

References

Bebb, O., et al. (2017). Performance of hospitals according to the ESC ACCA quality indicators and 30-day mortality for acute myocardial infarction: national cohort study using the United Kingdom Myocardial Ischaemia National Audit Project (MINAP) register. *Eur Heart J*, 38, 974–982.

Bowling, A. (2017). *Measuring Health* (4th edn). London: Open University Press.

Bray, B.D., et al. (2018). Socioeconomic disparities in first stroke incidence, quality of care, and survival: a nationwide registry-based cohort study of 44 million adults in England. *Lancet Public Health*, 3, e185–e193.

Campbell, M.J., Jacques, R.M., Fotheringham, J., Maheswaran, R., & Nicholl, J. (2012). Developing a summary hospital mortality index: retrospective analysis in English hospitals over five years. *BMJ*, 344, e1001.

Charlton, J.R., Hartley, R.M., Silver, R., & Holland, W.W. (1983). Geographical variation in mortality from conditions amenable to medical intervention in England and Wales. *Lancet*, 1(8326, Pt 1), 691–696.

Clark, D.M., Canvin, L., Green, J., Layard, R., Pilling, S., & Janecka, M. (2018). Transparency about the outcomes of mental health services (IAPT approach): an analysis of public data. *Lancet*, 391, 679–686.

Commonwealth Fund. (2011). *Why Not The Best? Results from the National Scorecare on US Health System Performance, 2011*. Washington, DC: Commonwealth Fund.

Cunningham, S.J., Garratt, A.M., & Hunt, N.P. (2000). Development of a condition-specific quality of life measure for patients with dentofacial deformity: I. Reliability of the instrument. *Community Dent Oral Epidemiol*, 28, 195–201.

Donabedian, A. (1966). Evaluating the quality of medical care. *Milbank Mem Fund Q*, 44, 166–206.

Donabedian, A. (2003). *An Introduction to Quality Assurance in Health Care*. Oxford, New York: Oxford University Press.

Dyer, C. (2001). Bristol inquiry condemns hospital's 'club culture'. *BMJ (Clin Res)*, 323, 181.

EuroQuol Group. (1990). EuroQol–a new facility for the measurement of health-related quality of life. *Health Policy*, 16, 199–208.

George, S., Read, S., Westlake, L., Williams, B., Fraser-Moodie, A., & Pritty, P. (1992). Evaluation of nurse triage in a British accident and emergency department. *BMJ*, 304, 876–878.

Goldstein, H. & Speigelhalter, D.J. (1996). League tables and their limitations: statistical issues in comparisons of institutional performance. *J Stat Soc Ser A*, 159, 385–443.

Greenhalgh, T., et al. (2018). Real-world implementation of video outpatient consultations at macro, meso, and micro levels: mixed-method study. *J Med Internet Res*, 20, e150.

Heslop, P., Blair, P., Fleming, P., Hoghton, M., Marriott, A., & Russ, L. (2013). *Confidential Inquiry into Premature Deaths of People with Learning Disabilities (CIPOLD) Final Report*. Bristol: CIPOLD. Available at: http://www.bristol.ac.uk/cipold/fullfinalreport.pdf [accessed 17 July 2019].

Hurwitz, B. & Vass, A. (2002). What's a good doctor and how can you make one. *BMJ*, 325, 667.

Illich, I. (1976). *Limits to Medicine. Medical Nemesis: The Expropriation of Health*. Harmondsworth: Penguin Books.

Kelley, E. & Hurst, J. (2006). *Health Care Quality Indicators Project Conceptual Framework Paper*. Paris: OECD. Available at: https://www.oecd.org/els/health-systems/36262363.pdf [accessed 17 July 2019].

Klein, M.W., Malone, M.F., Bennis, W.G., & Berkowitz, N.H. (1961). Problems of measuring patient care in the out-patient department. *J Health Hum Behav*, 2, 138–144.

Kohn, L.T., Corrigan, J., & Donaldson, M.S. (2000). *To Err Is Human: Building A Safer Health System*. Washington, DC: National Academy Press.

Kruk, M.E., Gage, A.D., Joseph, N.T., Danaei, G., García–Saisó, S., & Salomon, J.A. (2018). Mortality due to low-quality health systems in the universal health coverage era: a systematic analysis of amenable deaths in 137 countries. *Lancet*, 392, 2203–2212.

Kutz, T.L., Roszhart, J.M., Hale, M., Dolan, V., Suchomski, G., & Jaeger, C. (2018). Improving comprehensive care for patients with diabetes. *BMJ Open Qual*, 7, e000101.

Last, J.M. (2007). *A Dictionary of Public Health*. Oxford: Oxford University Press.

Lilford, R. & Pronovost, P. (2010). Using hospital mortality rates to judge hospital performance: a bad idea that just won't go away. *BMJ*, 340, c2016.

Lundgren–Nilsson, Å., et al. (2018). Patient-reported outcome measures in osteoarthritis: a systematic search and review of their use and psychometric properties. *RMD Open*, 4, e000715.

Masuy–Stroobant, G. & Gourbin, C. (1995). Infant health and mortality indicators: their accuracy for monitoring the socio-economic development in the Europe of 1994. *Eur J Popul*, 11, 63–84.

Maternal, Newborn and Infant Clinical Outcome Review Programme. (2014). *Saving Lives, Improving Mothers' Care: Lessons Learned to Inform Future Maternity Care from the UK and Ireland Confidential Enquiries into Maternal Deaths and Morbidity 2009–2012*. Oxford, National Perinatal Epidemiology Unit. Available at: https://www.npeu.ox.ac.uk/downloads/files/mbrrace-uk/reports/Saving%20Lives%20Improving%20Mothers%20Care%20report%202014%20Full.pdf [accessed 17 July 2019].

Maxwell, R.J. (1984). Quality assessment in health. *BMJ (Clin Res)*, 288, 1470–1472.

Newhouse, J.P. (2004). Consumer-directed health plans and the RAND Health Insurance Experiment. *Health Aff*, 23(6), 107–113.

Pemberton, J. & Cust, G. (1986). An epidemic of osteoporosis? *Community Med*, 8, 322–328.

Ramsay, J., Campbell, J.L., Schroter, S., Green, J., & Roland, M. (2000). The General Practice Assessment Survey (GPAS): tests of data quality and measurement properties. *Fam Pract*, 17, 372.

Rao, M., Clarke, A., Sanderson, C., & Hammersley, R. (2006). Patients' own assessments of quality of primary care compared with objective records based measures of technical quality of care: cross sectional study. *BMJ*, 333, 19.

Roland, M. (2004). Linking physicians' pay to the quality of care—a major experiment in the United Kingdom. *New Engl J Med*, 351(14), 1448–1454.

Starfield, B. (2000). Is US health really the best in the world? *JAMA*, 284(4), 483–485.

Streiner, D.L., Norman, G.R., & Cairney, J. (2014). *Health Measurement Scales. A Practical Guide to Their Development and Use* (5th edn). Oxford: Oxford University Press.

Ware, J.E., Bayliss, M.S., Rogers, W.H., Kosinski, M., & Tarlov, A.R. (1996). Differences in 4 year health outcomes for elderly and poor chronically ill patients treated in HMO and fee for service systems. *JAMA*, 276, 1039–1047.

12

Perspectives on healthcare quality and safety

Stephanie Russ and Nick Sevdalis

12.1 Introduction

Healthcare is characterized by the complexity of its processes. Most healthcare organizations fall under the umbrella term of 'complex systems', where there are many interacting parts (including people and technologies), each with their own degree of diversity. The challenge posed by such systems is that it is not always possible to predict the behaviour of the system based on knowledge of its components (World Health Organization, 2009). For example, if an elderly person experiences a hip fracture, her care will require coordination between multiple professionals from many different disciplines, including paramedics, radiologists, surgeons, anaesthetists, operating theatre staff, nurses, elderly care physicians, pharmacists, and rehabilitation experts. Feeding into this, services will also be required from device manufacturers and teams responsible for preparation of sterile supplies, hospital food, and hospital cleaning, among others. Additional factors surrounding her care will also vary depending on where and when she is treated, including contextual factors (e.g. staffing levels and distractions), technical factors (e.g. availability and reliability of equipment), and organizational factors (e.g. processes, procedures and culture). On top of this, each patient's condition, their risk factors, their comorbidities, and their resulting treatment requirements are unique; healthcare does not often produce standardized outputs and products like those of other industries. The complexity resulting from the interrelatedness of these components means that there are many opportunities for the quality of care to be compromised and for errors to arise, which can potentially impact on patients. Thus, healthcare, in common with other complex industries, is a high-risk activity.

This chapter discusses quality and safety in healthcare, drawing on material at the intersection of three novel scientific approaches, which have all developed in the past two decades (Figure 12.1). *Patient safety science* takes a scientific approach to the prevention, avoidance, and amelioration of adverse outcomes or injuries to patients stemming from the healthcare process (Vincent, 2010). *Improvement science* represents a scientific approach to achieving better patient experience and outcomes through changing provider behaviour and organization, using systematic change methods and strategies (Batalden & Davidoff, 2007). *Implementation science* represents the

Stephanie Russ and Nick Sevdalis, *Perspectives on healthcare quality and safety* In: *Healthcare Public Health*. Edited by: Martin Gulliford and Edmund Jessop, Oxford University Press (2020). © Oxford University Press. DOI: 10.1093/oso/9780198837206.003.0012.

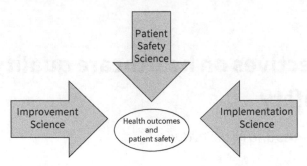

Figure 12.1 Intersection of three new sciences to improve healthcare quality and safety.

scientific study of methods to promote the uptake of research findings into routine healthcare practice or policy (Eccles & Mittman, 2006). We show how these three new applied health sciences can be employed to improve quality and safety, and achieve better health outcomes for patients.

12.2 Patient safety science

12.2.1 Definition and classification of patient safety problems

Far from being a vague concept, quality of care can now be precisely defined as 'the degree to which health services for individuals and populations increase the likelihood of desired health outcomes and are consistent with current professional knowledge' (Lohr, 1990). High-quality care should be safe and timely, as well as being effective, efficient, equitable, and patient-centred. Patient safety can be defined as 'the avoidance, prevention and amelioration of adverse outcomes or injuries stemming from the process of healthcare' (Vincent, 2010). An adverse event is 'an injury caused by medical management rather than the underlying condition of the patient', whereas an error is 'the failure of a planned action to be completed as intended' (error of execution) or 'the use of an inadequate plan to achieve an aim' (error of planning) (Kohn et al., 2000). An error has the potential to, but does not always, lead to harm. (See Box 12.1 for definitions of key concepts.)

Despite representing just one aspect of healthcare quality, patient safety has received a lot of attention in the research arena, as well as in the media, and represents a significant public health concern. This is largely due to the high frequency of adverse events in healthcare and the huge impact they have on people and organizations, explaining why the study of patient safety has emerged as a 'science' in its own right.

Studies carried out across a number of western healthcare systems report that around one in ten hospital inpatients suffers an adverse event. In the USA, this equates

---

Box 12.1 Key definitions

Quality: the degree to which health services for individuals and populations increase the likelihood of desired health outcomes and are consistent with current professional knowledge

High-quality care: care that is safe, timely, effective, efficient, patient-centred, and equitable

Quality improvement: better patient experience and outcomes achieved through changing provider behaviour and organization, through using a systematic change method and strategies

Patient safety: the avoidance, prevention, and amelioration of adverse outcomes or injuries stemming from the process of healthcare

Adverse event: an injury caused by medical management rather than the underlying condition of the patient

---

to some 44,000 to 98,000 people dying each year as a result of medical error (de Vries et al., 2008). This rate of adverse events is extremely high; healthcare is much less safe than industries that equally engage large numbers of people, such as travel by air or rail. The impact of such events can be catastrophic not only for the patient and their family, but also for the healthcare staff involved and for the healthcare organization as a whole (at both a reputational and financial level).

There are many different types of adverse events; those that are well studied to date are summarized in Box 12.2. Medication errors represent some of the best-studied problems in healthcare. Because of the tight regulation of drug marketing and prescription, errors of drug preparation, prescribing, and administration are possible to study from routinely collected data sources. The growing population of older people with multimorbidity has been associated with an increase in polypharmacy and increased risks of adverse drug reactions and drug–drug interactions. There has also been an increase in potentially inappropriate prescribing, which can be evaluated using standardized methods (O'Mahony et al., 2015).

Hospital-acquired infections (HAIs) represent another major concern. In the UK, 6–7% of patients will acquire a HAI, costing the NHS in excess of £1 billion annually (National Institute for Health and Care Excellence, 2016). These infections commonly result from invasive procedures and indwelling devices that may become contaminated, and are linked to factors such as length of hospital stay, avoidable hospital admissions, and antimicrobial resistance (National Institute for Health and Care Excellence, 2016). Antimicrobial resistance is increasing, to a large extent because of the unnecessary and inappropriate use of antibiotics in healthcare settings. Rates of some HAIs, such as MRSA infections, have declined rapidly as a result of control strategies, but other infections, such as gram-negative bloodstream infections, are increasing (Public Health England, 2017). Hospital hand-hygiene campaigns have shown the

---

Box 12.2 Types of well-studied errors and adverse events

Medication errors
  Prescribing; preparation
  Administration; adverse drug events

Hospital-acquired infection
  Indwelling devices
  Pneumonia; MRSA; C. Diff

Procedural adverse events
  Surgical-site infection
  Wrong site, patient, or procedure

Diagnostic errors
  Accuracy (misdiagnosis)
  Timing (diagnostic delay)

Documentation errors
  Missing record
  Inaccurate record

Communication errors
  Poor teamwork
  Lack of information flow

---

potential to dramatically reduce HAIs but depend on effective implementation of the campaigns themselves, and the process of behaviour and culture change, which is notoriously challenging (Lorencatto et al., 2018; Mackley et al., 2018).

Rates of adverse events tend to be higher in the context of surgical care than in other hospital specialties/departments (de Vries et al., 2008). Surgical procedures can be associated with infections but may also be complicated by a wider range of adverse events, including procedures being performed at the wrong site and surgical objects being retained in the body (see Section 12.2.2). Diagnostic errors tend to be underevaluated because they are difficult to study. Diagnostic errors are a particular concern to clinical practitioners, but health psychologists have also become interested in studying them because clinical diagnostic thinking is not always well evidenced-based and may rely on heuristics that are susceptible to bias, leading to faulty decision making.

Documentation errors arise if patients' notes are missing or incorrectly filed, or if notes are inadequate or not recorded correctly in the first place (Braff et al., 2011). In primary care, electronic health records are now well established, leading to generally better data recording. However, hospitals often rely on paper-based records that become increasingly bulky and hard to read as patients' journeys become more complex. Healthcare team working relies on communication between healthcare workers, and between healthcare workers and patients. Errors from failures of communication are particularly likely to occur at transitions in care. These include transitions between shift-working members of staff; between clinical teams, when children transition to adult services; and between healthcare organizational boundaries, when patients are transferred between healthcare facilities, or from healthcare to home (Cowie et al., 2009).

12.2.2 'Never' events

With awareness about the incidence and nature of medical error growing, we now recognize the existence of 'never' events—the kind of mistakes that should never happen in the field of medical care when best practices are being followed. These are serious incidents that are considered wholly preventable if the available preventive measures, such as national guidelines and mandatory procedures, are implemented and adhered to. In the UK, the list of 'never' events was revised in 2018 and now totals sixteen. These include the occurrence of surgery at the wrong site or on the wrong patient; having surgical instruments retained in the body after surgery; administration of medication by the wrong route; chest or neck entrapment in bed rails; and misplaced naso- or -oro-gastric tubes (NHS Improvement, 2018). The UK now requires mandatory reporting of 'never' events, but there is evidence that even these events are under-reported due to shifting definitions. Greater attention to the prevention of 'never' events is helping to reduce their occurrence (Wahid et al., 2016), yet in the USA, there are still 2,500 cases of wrong-site surgery per year out of 75 million procedures performed (0.0003%). If we compare this with the 10 million aircraft flights each year in the USA, this would be consistent with one flight crashing per day, a rate that would be considered wholly unacceptable.

12.2.3 Person-focused versus system-focused approaches in patient safety

Analysis of patient-safety incidents historically followed a 'person-focused' approach to error, which places the focus of error causation on the individual(s) involved. The assumption is that errors occur as a result of deficiencies in human mental processes and behaviours which are under an individual's control, for example, carelessness or inattention. As such, responses to error also focus on the individual, aiming to reduce unwanted variation in such processes/behaviours, for example through retraining, but often, in more serious cases, including the attribution of blame and the initiation of disciplinary processes. Over time, the primary focus has shifted to the roles of healthcare systems, with the perception that adverse events are the product of defective systems and that the context within which we work increases vulnerability towards error. This 'system-focused' approach recognizes that the human actors within systems are necessarily error-prone because of their human capabilities (humans are, and always will be, fallible). The response to error becomes focused on identifying and correcting weaknesses within the system, thus making it easier for humans to 'do the right thing' (Reason, 2000).

The 'person' approach and the 'system' approach to patient safety can be viewed as the poles of a continuum which is reflected in the safety culture of an organization. A culture that seeks to apportion blame to individuals stands in contrast to a culture which focuses on how to improve systems to reduce the potential for human errors and their associated impacts. Different hospitals may take differing positions on this continuum, and different services within the same hospital may also differ in their approach, which may also fluctuate over time and be responsive to how major incidents are handled and dealt with.

This debate concerning the relative roles of people and systems relates to the concept of healthcare as a complex 'socio-technical system' (Figure 12.2). The healthcare system includes a social component consisting of individual human actors (healthcare workers) who have to complete a variety of evidence-based tasks. To do these tasks, they draw on technology and tools including diagnostic aids, clinical guidelines, and treatment options. This work is conducted within a physical environment, such as a hospital building or general practice premises, that may not always be optimally

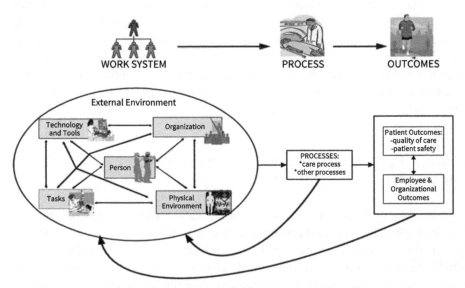

Figure 12.2 Healthcare as a 'socio-technical' system.

designed for its present use, and within the context of an organization that arranges and controls the individual elements. This reinforces the concept that errors occur as a result of interacting failures within multiple components of the system. It shows how changes within any one component might influence performance in other, potentially far-reaching areas (Carayon et al., 2006).

12.2.4 Risk management

In the 'system' approach, patient-safety incidents represent a failure of risk management. While the proximal causes of adverse events may be an active error on the part of a healthcare worker, the underlying or root causes are the latent error-producing conditions, or hazards, in the local workplace or wider organization that allowed that unsafe act to occur. This is the basis of a framework for understanding healthcare incidents that has attracted significant attention in the past two decades: psychologist James Reason's 'Swiss cheese' model of organizational accidents. If there are gaps in risk control at several levels of the organization, these gaps can become aligned so that hazards are transmitted from one level to the next, ultimately allowing a serious incident to occur.

The 'Swiss cheese' model (see Figure 12.3) emphasizes the need to create systems that are better able to tolerate and contain the effects of error by building in defences at each level of the system, to provide safeguards against hazards, so they do not propagate within the system and result in harm (Reason, 2000, 2006, 2016). High-quality health systems should be designed to ensure that risks are mitigated before any patient-safety incident occurs. 'Perfect' risk-management strategies

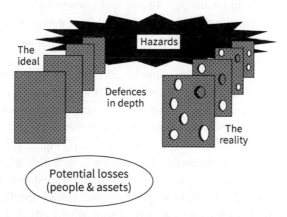

Figure 12.3 James Reason's 'Swiss cheese' model. The reality being that all systems will have gaps/holes in their risk control at multiple levels—and we should look to plug these holes to improve a system's defences against safety incidents.

are difficult (if not impossible) to design for healthcare environments due to their complexity, but various approaches are available, ranging from physical barriers (e.g. a locked cupboard or the use of unique syringe adaptors to prevent wrong-route drug administration) through to policies and procedures to encourage safe working practices, improved teamwork, appropriate supervision, and education and training.

12.2.5 Human factors

Highlighting the importance of taking a systems rather than a person approach to safety is not to deny the importance of human behaviour and performance in the safe delivery of care—quite the opposite. 'Human factors' science is a leading approach in the understanding of how to make systems safer in a range of safety-critical industries. In healthcare, human factors science allows us to 'enhance clinical performance through an understanding of the effects of teamwork, tasks, equipment, workspace, culture and organisation on human behaviour and abilities and apply that knowledge in clinical settings' (Catchpole, 2012). By taking this approach, we can better understand how to intervene and make improvements to the system which are most likely to increase the occurrence of safe human behaviours. In the same vein, by acknowledging human limitations, human factors science offers ways to minimize and mitigate human frailties, so reducing medical error and its consequences.

A central tenet of the human factors approach is the recognition that, at an individual and team level, effective clinical performance is not only a product of technical skill and knowledge but is highly dependent on the quality of non-technical skills. Non-technical skills are the 'cognitive, social and personal resource skills that complement technical skills and contribute to safe and efficient task performance' (Flin & O'Connor, 2017). These non-technical skills include communication, decision making, situation awareness, leadership, stress and fatigue management, and workload management.

There is now strong evidence demonstrating a link between failures in non-technical skills and the occurrence of adverse events (Greenberg et al., 2007; Hull et al., 2012). This has led to the uptake of team-training programmes based around the crew-resource management techniques used in the aviation industry which are designed to promote and improve non-technical skills (Hughes et al., 2016; Neily et al., 2010). Such training represents one approach to building defences into a healthcare system: for example, increasing situation awareness may allow an individual to capture a hazard before it propagates to result in an error. Following initial application and spread through interventional specialties in healthcare (including obstetrics, anaesthesia, and surgery), non-technical skills training is becoming embedded across all healthcare specialties (e.g. Ellis & Sevdalis, 2019) and efforts are made to teach non-technical skills within the medical school curriculum (e.g. Hamilton et al., 2019).

12.2.6 Incident analysis

Incident analysis in healthcare is an essential element of risk management. It is a specialized and complex task, where the aim is to identify the underlying systems failures that led to an error, to learn from these, and to reduce risk by making improvements to prevent reoccurrence—not to apportion blame. Thus, the main goal of analysing an incident is to learn and improve. Numerous approaches have been reported in the healthcare evidence base and are currently applied, to allow such learning to take place. These include incident analysis itself, but also voluntary and mandatory incident reporting systems, mortality and morbidity reviews/conferences, analysis of claims/complaints data, and other methods (de Feijter et al., 2013).

Perhaps the most widely deployed approach to incident analysis in healthcare is root-cause analysis (RCA). RCA is a structured, retrospective investigation process that utilizes a set of tools and techniques informed by the concepts of human factors. It examines multiple system-level vulnerabilities as contributory factors themselves (i.e. not a single cause), and also looks at the interactions between them. RCA consists of a number of steps. The first step is to gather information from a range of sources and stakeholders (including the patient/family) and produce a detailed timeline of events leading up to the incident or error. Next, care-delivery problems are identified (i.e. what went wrong in the provision of care). These might include omissions such as a failure to monitor, observe, or act, or not seeking help when necessary, or wrong actions such as slips in the delivery of care. Following this, a detailed analysis consisting of a series of 'how' and 'why' questions is conducted, often aided by a RCA tool, to identify the associated contributory factors and root causes. Solutions, recommendations, and an action plan will then be generated and compiled into a report to be shared with the wider organization, the regulatory authority and the patient or their family. Recommendations and actions should be linked to specific root causes and prioritized, and a plan for their implementation should be made, including a timeline and identification of accountable individuals (Joint Commission, 2015).

A number of tools have been developed to assist in the process of RCA, specifically when it comes to identifying contributory factors and root causes that exacerbate care-delivery problems. Vincent's London Protocol, which is more than 20 years old but still in wide use, is an example of such a tool which draws on the 'Swiss cheese' model reviewed earlier in this chapter (Figure 12.4).[1] The London Protocol makes explicit, and brings to the fore, latent factors that might otherwise be overlooked. It

---

[1] A newer addition to the healthcare incident-analysis armoury is the Yorkshire Contributory Factors Framework, development of which was based on a review of studies focusing on the causes of hospital patient-safety incidents (Lawton et al., 2012). Regardless of the specific tool used, implementation of root-cause analysis in a manner focused on learning, and not blame, is a key factor for healthcare providers to engage meaningfully with it, so that the organization or service learn and avoid repeating similar failures in the future (Archer et al., 2017).

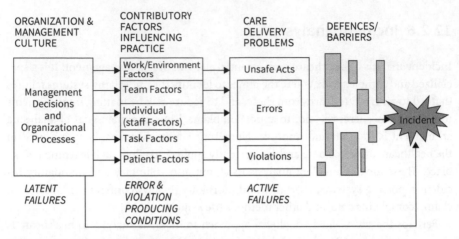

Figure 12.4 The London Protocol for incident analysis.

Reproduced with permission from Taylor–Adams, S. & Vincent, C., 'Systems analysis of clinical incidents: the London protocol'. *Clinical Risk*, Vol. 10, Issue 6, pp. 211–220. Copyright © 2004 SAGE Publications.

encourages the identification of contributory factors and root causes at various different levels of the system including:

Patient factors: for example, condition; language and communication; personality and social factors

Task and technology factors: for example, task design and clarity of structure; availability and use of protocols; availability and accuracy of test results; decision-making aids

Individual (staff) factors: for example, knowledge and skills; competence; physical and mental health

Team factors: for example, verbal and written communication; supervision and seeking help; team structure (congruence, consistency, leadership, etc.)

Work and environment factors: for example, staffing levels and skills mix; workload and shift patterns; design, availability, and maintenance of equipment; administrative and managerial support; environment

Organizational and management factors: for example, financial resources and constraints; organizational structure; policy, standards, and goals; safety culture and priorities

Institutional context factors: for example, economic and regulatory context; NHS executive; links with external organizations

12.3 Improvement science and quality improvement

12.3.1 Improvement science

Twenty years ago, major publications in the USA (*To Err is Human*; Kohn et al., 2000) and in the UK (*An Organization with a Memory*: Department of Health, 2000), based on data collected and analysed during the 1980s and 1990s, brought the issue of patient safety onto the policy agenda. These reports highlighted the incidence of the patient-safety problem as an epidemiological phenomenon, which required urgent attention and intervention. The scale of the problem (one in ten inpatients suffering an adverse event; Vincent et al., 2001) suggested this was a public health concern. This had the subsequent effect of triggering significant research and development investment in major healthcare economies globally (e.g. the Patient Safety Research Programme in the UK), aimed at understanding safety problems in depth so that improvement solutions and interventions could be designed, tested, and implemented at scale. This development ultimately drove the establishment of 'improvement science' (Berwick, 2008). The aim of 'improvement science' is to take a scientific approach to achieving better patient experience and outcomes through changing provider behaviour and organization, using systematic change methods and strategies (Batalden & Davidoff, 2007). Alongside its scientific development, over the past 20 years improvement science has permeated the world of healthcare at a practical level. Most, if not all, hospitals and other healthcare providers in advanced economies have quality-improvement departments and personnel specializing in improvement techniques. The approaches used in today's improvement science date back almost 100 years and are often identified with Walter Shewhart, William Edwards Deming, and Joseph Juran, who all worked to quality assure industrial manufacturing processes through the use of standardized tools and measurements (Varkey, 2007; Perla et al., 2013). Through their work, some of the well-known tools used by healthcare organizations today were first developed and applied, including the globally known Plan–Do–Study–Act (PDSA) cycle. Techniques such as the PDSA were the focus of the Institute for Healthcare Improvement (IHI), which was founded in 1991 to promote quality improvement in healthcare through dissemination and advocacy for these techniques, and also capacity development of the healthcare workforce and its leadership through an expansive training programme. The IHI's work has contributed significantly to the spread and adoption of improvement science within healthcare organizations, largely through the development and dissemination of its Model for Improvement (MfI).

12.3.2 Model for Improvement

The MfI breaks down the improvement process into three questions:

1. *What we are trying to achieve?* This question focuses on setting specific and achievable goals for improvement, which are designed to address problems identified in the delivery of care and should also be assessable.
2. *How will we know that a change is actually an improvement?* This question focuses on the importance of gathering appropriate data that allow a service to determine whether their efforts have resulted in improvement, and by how much.
3. *What changes can we make that will actually result in improvement?* This final question focuses on the process of developing, implementing, and evaluating improvement solutions and interventions within a service/organization.

The MfI proceeds through the application of the PDSA methodology. Initially, an intervention to be implemented is planned, in accordance with the improvement goal (Plan). The intervention (improvement change) is then implemented, typically at small scale (e.g. within one department or on one ward), to test whether it is workable and feasible to deliver in practice, and to allow it to introduce its effects (Do). The outcome of the intervention is subsequently studied by measuring the pre-agreed outcomes and assessing its impact on the service (Study). If the quality-improvement intervention is successful, the action plan should be full implementation at scale (Act). If results do not achieve intended outcomes, then further PDSA cycles follow (hence the intervention is cyclical).

12.3.3 Supporting principles

A number of principles support the application of improvement approaches such as the MfI. One such principle is that reliable and valid data-collection processes should be in place in order to provide baseline measurements of care quality and their changes over time, otherwise it is not possible to evaluate what impact, if any, an improvement intervention may have. Measurement for improvement is not quite the same as measurement for research: the aim is not to arrive at generalizations about a phenomenon but, rather, to offer a useful depiction of service parameters that require attention, including their baseline and post-intervention values. This allows stakeholders of the improvement process to evaluate whether a solution is working or whether further intervention development is required. Therefore, a related principle is that stakeholders ought to be engaged and involved in the improvement process from a very early stage: improvement is done with and not to healthcare providers. Technically, engagement allows providers to identify the metrics that are relevant to them and to offer their tacit knowledge regarding aspects of their services that require redevelopment or substantial change. Motivationally, this fosters a shared commitment and enthusiasm for changes to services. Establishing a patient group to offer a patient or service-user perspective on services is important because patients directly experience healthcare and have considerable knowledge to bring to the process of improvement.

A further related principle is that for improvement to work, deep understanding of a service or organizational configuration is necessary; after all, one cannot improve what one does not understand. To achieve this, part of the improvement process ought to involve detailed analysis of the care pathways that are to be improved. This is often done through techniques such as process mapping, which provide detailed description of an entire care pathway, so that the application of an improvement intervention can be planned precisely.

Lastly, quality improvement should aim to improve the reliability of care. Interventions should not be 'one-off' improvements but should ensure that care is error-free and consistent over time—hence of high reliability.

12.3.4 Limitations

Readers with epidemiological training will immediately identify limitations of the PDSA approach, including the possible lack of sample-size calculation and comparator groups in the traditional approach of large-scale healthcare research. However, one should consider the aims of improvement and juxtapose them to the aims of research. A formal research trial might take several years (and significant financial and human resources) to complete, and this is not usually a relevant timeline for quality-improvement interventions, where time is pressing and funds are limited to service funds, without the additional research and development funding which is typical of a trial. It follows that in the context of improvement science, measurement is considered to be an improvement activity rather than a research activity. Hence, data collection for improvement purposes is focused on putting knowledge into practice, and is often conducted at small scale and over short time-periods, with the aim of gaining enough information to learn confidently rather than being based on formal assessment of statistical power. The outcomes for improvement science evaluations often include process measures that evaluate whether the components of a system are performing as planned, as well as implementation outcomes such as fidelity, coverage, and feasibility (see Section 12.4.4). It is also important to consider and measure possible unintended consequences of improvement interventions, sometimes referred to as balancing measures. For example, an intervention to reduce length of stay might result in an increased number of readmissions, due to the early discharge of patients who then represent at the emergency department.

It should also be noted that carrying out improvement interventions and studies competently requires in-depth understanding of the MfI, PDSA, and other techniques. Despite the seeming simplicity of such approaches as the PDSA and related methods, or perhaps because of it, implementation of the techniques has, to date, been far from optimal: fidelity to the techniques has been low and patchy (Nicolay et al., 2012; Taylor et al., 2014). Training in improvement-science methods and specific improvement techniques is thus strongly required for the user to be able to apply them with competence, as intended.

12.4 Implementing patient safety solutions and improving care: the role of implementation science

12.4.1 The second translational gap

Prior to the twentieth century, medicine was generally ineffective and the few simple interventions available had considerable capacity to do harm (Wooton, 2006; Illich, 1976). We are now in an era where medicine and healthcare are continuously generating complex new evidence concerning the effectiveness and safety of medical interventions (e.g. new treatments, practical interventions, guidelines, policies, new technologies). Effective translation of this research into practice is necessary for the benefits to care to be realized, but there has been growing concern about the efficiency and effectiveness of research translation since the 1990s. In practice, evidence does not readily make its way into routine clinical care, despite the demonstration of benefits for patients; often there may be a significant time delay before evidence is taken up by healthcare practitioners. Additionally, interventions that appear to be effective in small-scale pilot studies fail to live up to expectations when rolled out in national strategies or fail to transfer from one country to another as a result of contextual differences. (See Box 12.3 for an example relating to the implementation of the WHO Surgical Safety Checklist in UK hospitals.)

Box 12.3 The WHO Surgical Safety Checklist: a case study for the need for implementation science

The WHO Surgical Safety Checklist was first reported in 2009 as a simple, inexpensive intervention for improving the care and reducing the risk of errors and injuries in patients undergoing surgery. In the initial evaluation, use of the checklist was associated with a 36% reduction in major complications, a 48% reduction in post-operative infections, and a 47% reduction in mortality (Haynes et al., 2009). Based on these results, the Department of Health in England made use of the checklist mandatory for hospitals in the NHS—and many other countries and healthcare systems globally did the same. However, a later large-scale evaluation across over 215,000 electronic patient records in Canada showed no effect from systematic use of the checklist in Ontario hospitals (Urbach et al., 2014). The lack of effect was hypothesized to be caused by an implementation gap, with the checklist being incompletely implemented by those charged with using it.

In a UK study of 565 patients, we found that, on average, only two thirds of the items on the checklist were checked, team members were absent in over 40% of cases, and they failed to pause or focus on the checks in more than 70% of cases (Russ et al., 2015a). Further qualitative research showed that checklist implementation varied greatly between and within hospitals, ranging from preplanned and phased approaches to the checklist simply 'appearing' in operating rooms, or staff feeling it had been imposed. The barriers to implementation of the checklist included problematic integration into pre-existing processes. The most common barrier was resistance from senior clinicians, indicating the need to foster strong leadership at a senior level and to instil accountability (Russ et al., 2015b).

Failures of implementation can be costly because of the resources wasted on interventions that are not fully utilized; failures of implementation also lead to loss of potential effectiveness. It is relevant to note that, in the UK, wrong-site surgery remains the most frequently notified 'never' event to date, in spite of the intended implementation of the surgical checklist which, amongst other goals, aims to eliminate wrong-site and wrong-person surgeries.

This disconnection between the development of interventions in research and their successful translation to clinical practice is the so-called 'second translational gap' (Pearson et al., 2012). The first translational gap is between basic science discoveries and translation into potential therapeutic interventions.

One of the barriers to the effective and rapid translation of evidence is that it is often generated in the special circumstances of a randomized controlled trial, or an otherwise controlled research setting, with carefully selected patients, by staff who have a high level of expertise in a given condition and its treatment, employing dedicated research funds and treatment facilities. This contrasts with the setting of widespread adoption into health services, where interventions need to be delivered by staff with often generalist training and expertise, with differing priorities and perspectives, to patients with a wider range of ages and comorbidities, and with more limited funds for service delivery. The fact that interventions are rarely, if ever, implemented as designed is a problem, because variability in implementation has been consistently shown to predict variability in outcomes. One approach to bridging the gap between research and practice is to collect 'real-world' evidence through trials that adopt a pragmatic perspective and test interventions in the circumstances in which they will eventually be adopted (Ford & Norrie, 2016). This, and other approaches that might aid the effective uptake of research findings, is the focus of implementation scientists.

12.4.2 The goals of implementation science

Implementation scientists are interested in understanding how best to promote the uptake of research findings into routine healthcare in clinical, organizational, or policy contexts. The establishment of the field of implementation science as an autonomous area of applied health research, complementary to those of patient safety and improvement sciences, is often taken to be 2006, when the first-ever peer-reviewed journal dedicated to this area was launched (*Implementation Science*), although implementation studies were carried out before then across all fields of healthcare and medicine. The field grew following the wave of the evidence-based medicine (EBM) movement in medicine and public health, with the ensuing frustration of many clinical and health scientists who saw interventions and programmes being well evidenced, yet their uptake within routine services remaining low. One study estimated the time lag between health evidence being produced and implemented routinely to be 17 years (Morris et al., 2011). This figure is quoted regularly to explain the need for a science of intervention implementation in health services and public health.

The specific aims and objectives of implementation science research include:

- Facilitating the widespread adoption of strategies for improving health-related processes and outcomes.
- Advancing knowledge on how best to replicate intervention effects in real-world settings.

- Understanding the aetiology of gaps between expected results and observed outcomes.
- Producing generalizable knowledge from insights regarding implementation processes, barriers, facilitators, and strategies.
- Developing, testing, and refining implementation theories and hypotheses, methods and measures.

Implementation scientists ask questions such as: Why do interventions work in one setting but not in another? Why do interventions display unintended effects? Why do interventions lose effectiveness over months or years of implementation?

12.4.3 Implementation frameworks and strategies

Implementation science increasingly calls on theoretical approaches to provide better understanding and explanation of how and why implementation succeeds or fails. Implementation studies now apply theories borrowed from disciplines such as psychology, sociology, and organizational theory. Theories, models, and frameworks have also emerged from within implementation science itself. Due to the large number of theories, models, and frameworks that have been developed and applied to the field of implementation science, the terms are often used interchangeably, with confusion around which one to apply to get the best out of one's implementation efforts. However, implementation theories, models, and frameworks have a number of shared objectives, which are to aid:

- Describing and/or guiding the process of translating research into practice.
- Understanding and/or explaining what influences implementation outcomes.
- Evaluating implementation.

Using a theoretical framework or model to guide implementation research will allow results to be more reliably generalized and built upon across studies and contexts (Nilsen, 2015; Tabak et al., 2012).

The Consolidated Framework for Implementation Research (CFIR) is an example of an implementation science framework that can be used to guide implementation research. The CFIR draws on elements from 19 different implementation theories and frameworks, and integrates them into a single taxonomy for exploring the effectiveness of implementation within a given context (Damschroder et al., 2009; Kirk et al., 2015; Palinkas et al., 2015). The CFIR comprises 39 constructs, organized across five major domains, all of which interact to influence implementation effectiveness. These include factors related to the intervention itself (intervention); factors external to the organization implementing the intervention (outer setting); characteristics of that organization (inner setting); characteristics of the individuals involved in implementing the intervention (individuals); and the process of implementation (process) (Figure 12.5.) The CFIR

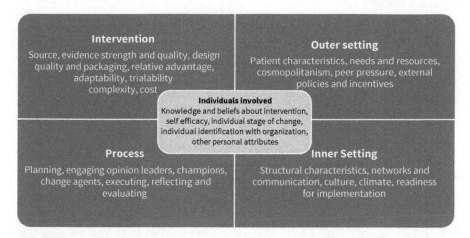

Intervention
Source, evidence strength and quality, design quality and packaging, relative advantage, adaptability, trialability complexity, cost

Outer setting
Patient characteristics, needs and resources, cosmopolitanism, peer pressure, external policies and incentives

Individuals involved
Knowledge and beliefs about intervention, self efficacy, individual stage of change, individual identification with organization, other personal attributes

Process
Planning, engaging opinion leaders, champions, change agents, executing, reflecting and evaluating

Inner Setting
Structural characteristics, networks and communication, culture, climate, readiness for implementation

Figure 12.5 The Consolidated Framework for Implementation Research.

provides a common language for researchers to use when referring to implementation concepts, and a standardized list of constructs to guide the identification of variables which are most likely to be salient to implementation. It can be used to help develop a methodological approach to assessing implementation, as well as to guide the analysis, interpretation, and reporting of findings.

CFIR is therefore a good example of a practical framework for patient safety and improvement scientists and practitioners tasked with improving a service via implementation of an evidenced practice (e.g. the WHO checklist), or even with maintaining successful uptake of the practice over time since original implementation. Implementation frameworks thus do not replace or negate the need for safety and improvement frameworks; they work to complement them, to support their application with high fidelity of improvement solutions, and to help explain why and when such application may be problematic or ineffective.

Implementation frameworks such as CFIR allow the identification of potential barriers to the implementation of an improvement intervention, which then require addressing. This is achieved via a number of implementation strategies, which are methods or techniques used to enhance the adoption, implementation, and sustainability of a clinical programme, practice, or intervention (Proctor et al., 2013). Single implementation strategies may be used (e.g. a single education programme), but implementation efforts are likely to be most successful when using a range of strategies (i.e. a multifaceted approach). Recent research has identified nine categories with over 70 discrete implementation strategies of relevance to healthcare researchers, practitioners, and policy makers (Powell et al., 2015) (Box 12.4).

Choosing the best implementation strategies for any given improvement effort is important for its success. Implementation strategies should be matched to the barriers and facilitators surrounding the implementation of a new process change or evidence-based practice. For example, if one barrier to implementation of an intervention is a

---

Box 12.4   Categories of implementation strategy

Evaluative and iterative strategies: for example, assess readiness for change and identify barriers and facilitators; audit and provide feedback

Provide iterative assistance: for example, provide clinical supervision and training; facilitate with interactive problem solving and support

Adapt and tailor to context: for example, promote adaptability of the intervention; tailor strategies to address barriers and leverage facilitators

Develop stakeholder interrelationships: for example, identify and prepare champions; inform local-opinion leaders

Train and educate stakeholders: for example, conduct ongoing training; distribute educational materials

Support clinicians: for example, provide reminders to prompt use of the intervention; revise professional roles

Engage patients and service users: for example, intervene with patients to enhance uptake and adherence; use mass media

Utilize financial strategies: for example, alter incentive/allowance structures; develop disincentives

Change infrastructure: for example, mandate the change; change liability laws

---

lack of knowledge/skills, then one appropriate implementation strategy would be the distribution of educational materials. On the other hand, if one facilitator to implementation is that certain individuals are motivated and committed to implementing an intervention, then one appropriate implementation strategy would be to recruit these individuals as clinical champions to drive uptake amongst colleagues. Detailed work with stakeholders and a good understanding of the context within which the safety or other improvement intervention is aimed, through frameworks such as CFIR, facilitate the selection of appropriate strategies (Powell et al., 2017).

12.4.4   The concept of implementation outcomes

Once an improvement intervention of evidenced practice has been implemented using the chosen implementation strategies, there is a need to gauge whether or not implementation has been successful. Implementation outcomes serve as indicators or measures of implementation success. Proctor et al. (2011), using evidence review and synthesis and expert consensus methodologies, produced a working taxonomy of eight conceptually distinct implementation outcomes that can be assessed to better understand the extent and effectiveness of implementation. These range from understanding the perceived acceptability of the improvement to measuring whether the improvement is being used with fidelity (i.e. how it was intended to be used) (Table 12.1).

Table 12.1 Implementation outcomes

Implementation outcome	Definition
Acceptability	Perception amongst stakeholders that new intervention is agreeable
Adoption	Intention to apply or application of new intervention
Appropriateness	Perceived relevance of intervention to a setting, audience, or problem
Feasibility	Extent to which an intervention can be applied
Fidelity	Extent to which an intervention is applied as originally designed/intended
Implementation costs	Costs of the delivery strategy, including the costs of the intervention itself
Coverage	Extent to which eligible patients/population actually receive intervention
Sustainability	Extent to which a new intervention becomes routinely available/is maintained post introduction

While we now agree on what outcomes are important to measure, there is less consensus around the scales or instruments we should use to measure them. A systematic review in the context of mental health revealed that over 104 different instruments had been used to capture the outcomes (with the majority assessing acceptability and adoption), with generally poor psychometric properties (Lewis et al., 2015). Recent research is attempting therefore to develop standardized scales to capture implementation outcomes, to bring consistency and comparability to the field (e.g. Khadjesari et al., 2017; Weiner et al., 2017).

12.5 Conclusion

In this chapter, we offer an introduction to the recently developed applied health science fields of patient safety, improvement, and implementation sciences. The quest to improve quality and safety in healthcare can be best achieved by combining approaches and guiding principles from these different fields. Developed over the past two decades, they each have an important role to play in improving care-delivery processes and pathways, and hence the outcomes of healthcare that are received and experienced by patients and service users. Problems in the delivery of healthcare, identified for the first time 20 years ago, now have well-established solutions; and numerous techniques have been adapted and subsequently adopted within healthcare which originated in other industries—from manufacturing to aviation.

In 2019, the Global Ministerial Summit for Patient Safety issued the Jeddah Declaration that explicitly stated that 'to transform patient safety over the next 20 years, it is imperative that healthcare systems focus on implementation strategies to reduce the so called "2nd translational gap", thereby maximizing the added value of the expansive evidence base on patient safety' (Global Ministerial Summit for Patient Safety, 2019). Modern public health therefore needs to reap the benefits of the ever-expanding multidisciplinary space of these newly emerged sciences to address the burden of adverse events and harm that is due to the delivery of healthcare—which impacts on large numbers of patients and their families, as well as providers and the system of healthcare as a whole. The readers of this book are ideally placed to embrace the available scientific knowledge and use it to improve health services' safety outcomes, nationally and globally.

References

Archer, S., et al. (2017). Development of a theoretical framework of factors affecting patient safety incident reporting: a theoretical review of the literature. *BMJ Open*, 7, e017155.

Batalden, P.B. & Davidoff, F. (2007). What is 'quality improvement' and how can it transform healthcare? *Qual Saf Health Care*, 16, 2–3.

Berwick, B.M. (2008). The science of improvement. *JAMA*, 299, 1182–1184.

Braaf, S., Manias, E., & Riley, R. (2011). The role of documents and documentation in communication failure across the perioperative pathway. A literature review. *Int J Nurs Stud*, 48, 1024–1038.

Carayon, P., Xie, A., & Kianfar, S. (2014). Human factors and ergonomics as a patient safety practice. *BMJ Qual Saf*, 23(3), 196–205.

Carayon, P., et al. (2006). Work system design for patient safety: the SEIPS model. *Qual Saf Health Care*, 15(suppl 1), i50–58.

Catchpole K. Cited in department of health human factors reference group interim report, 1 March 2012, National Quality Board. March 2012. http://www.england.nhs.uk/ourwork/part-rel/nqb/ag-min/ (Accessed 05.03.2020)

Cowie, L., Morgan, M., White, P., & Gulliford, M. (2009). Experience of continuity of care of patients with multiple long-term conditions in England. *J Health Serv Res Policy*, 14, 82–87.

Damschroder, L.J., Aron, D.C., Keith, R.E., Kirsh, S.R., Alexander, J.A., & Lowery, J.C. (2009). Fostering implementation of health services research findings into practice: a consolidated framework for advancing implementation science. *Implement Sci*, 4(1), 50.

de Feijter, J.M., de Grave, W.S., Koopmans, R.P., & Scherpbier, A.J. (2013). Informal learning from error in hospitals: what do we learn, how do we learn and how can informal learning be enhanced? A narrative review. *Adv Health Sci Educ Theory Pract*, 18(4), 787–805.

Department of Health. (2000). *An Organisation with a Memory*. London: Department of Health.

de Vries, E.N., Ramrattan, M.A., Smorenburg, S.M., Gouma, D.J., & Boermeester, M.A. (2008). The incidence and nature of in-hospital adverse events: a systematic review. *BMJ Qual Saf*, 17(3), 216–223.

Eccles, M.P. & Mittman, B.S. (2006). Welcome to implementation science. *Implement Sci*, 1, 1.

Ellis, G. & Sevdalis, N. (2019). Understanding and improving multidisciplinary team working in geriatric medicine. *Age Ageing*, 48(4), 498–505. doi: 10.1093/ageing/afz021

Flin, R. & O'Connor, P. (2017). *Safety at the Sharp End: A Guide to Non-Technical Skills.* CRC Press.

Ford, I. & Norrie, J. (2016). Pragmatic trials. *New Engl J Med*, 375(5), 454–463.

Global Ministerial Summit on Patient Safety. (2019). *Jeddah Declaration on Patient Safety*. Available at: https://www.bundesgesundheitsministerium.de/fileadmin/Dateien/3_Downloads/P/Patientensicherheit/PSS_2019/Patientensicherheit_Erklaerung_Dschidda_2019.pdf [accessed 21 July 2019].

Greenberg, C.C., et al. (2007). Patterns of communication breakdowns resulting in injury to surgical patients. *J Am Coll Surg*, 204(4), 533–540.

Hamilton, A.L., Kerins, J., MacCrossan, M.A., & Tallentire, V.R. (2019). Medical students' non-technical skills (Medi-StuNTS): preliminary work developing a behavioural marker system for the non-technical skills of medical students in acute care. *BMJ Simul Technol Enhanc Learn*, 5, 130–139.

Haynes, A.B., et al. (2009). A surgical safety checklist to reduce morbidity and mortality in a global population. *New Engl J Med*, 360(5), 491–499.

Hughes, A.M., et al. (2016). Saving lives: a meta-analysis of team training in healthcare. *J Appl Psychol*, 101(9), 1266.

Hull, L., Arora, S., Aggarwal, R., Darzi, A., Vincent, C., & Sevdalis, N. (2012). The impact of nontechnical skills on technical performance in surgery: a systematic review. *J Am Coll Surg*, 214(2), 214–230.

Illich, I. (1976). *Limits to Medicine. Medical Nemesis: The Expropriation of Health.* Harmondsworth: Penguin Books.

Joint Commission. (2015). *Root Cause Analysis in Healthcare: Tools and Techniques*. Oak Brook, Illinois: Joint Commission Resources. Available at: https://www.jcrinc.com/assets/1/14/EBRCA15Sample.pdf

Khadjesari, Z., Vitoratou, S., Sevdalis, N., & Hull, L. (2017). Implementation outcome assessment instruments used in physical healthcare settings and their measurement properties: a systematic review protocol. *BMJ Open*, 7(10), e017972.

Kirk, M.A., Kelley, C., Yankey, N., Birken, S.A., Abadie, B., & Damschroder, L. (2015). A systematic review of the use of the consolidated framework for implementation research. *Implement Sci*, 11, 72.

Kohn, L.T., Corrigan, J.M., & Donaldson, M.S. (2000). *To Err Is Human*. Washington, DC: Institute of Medicine.

Lawton, R., McEachan, R.R., Giles, S.J., Sirriyeh, R., Watt, I.S., & Wright, J. (2012). Development of an evidence-based framework of factors contributing to patient safety incidents in hospital settings: a systematic review. *BMJ Qual Saf*, 21(5), 369–80.

Lewis, C.C., Fischer, S., Weiner, B.J., Stanick, C., Kim, M., & Martinez, R.G. (2015). Outcomes for implementation science: an enhanced systematic review of instruments using evidence-based rating criteria. *Implement Sci*, 10, 155.

Lohr KNf ed. Medicare: A Strategy for Quality Assurance, v I. Washington, DC: National Academy Pr; 1990:21.

Lorencatto, F., Charani, E., Sevdalis, N., Tarrant, C., & Davey, P. (2018). Driving sustainable change in antimicrobial prescribing practice: how can social and behavioural sciences help? *J Antimicrob Chemother*, 73(10), 2613–2624.

Mackley, A., Baker, C., & Bate, A. (2018). *Raising Standards of Infection Prevention and Control in the NHS*. London: House of Commons Library. Available at: https://researchbriefings.files.parliament.uk/documents/CDP-2018-0116/CDP-2018-0116.pdf

Morris, Z.S., Wooding, S., & Grant, J. (2011). The answer is 17 years, what is the question: understanding time lags in translational research. *J R Soc Med*, 104(12), 510–520.

National Institute for Health and Care Excellence. (2016). *Healthcare-Acquired Infections.* London: National Institute for Health and Care Excellence. Available at: https://www.nice.org.uk/guidance/qs113/resources/healthcareassociated-infections-pdf-75545296430533

Neily, J., et al. (2010). Association between implementation of a medical team training program and surgical mortality. *JAMA*, 304(15), 1693–1700.

NHS Improvement. (2018). Never Events List. Available at: https://improvement.nhs.uk/documents/2899/Never_Events_list_2018_FINAL_v7.pdf

Nicolay, C.R., et al. (2012). Systematic review of the application of the plan-do-study-act method to improve quality in healthcare. *Br J Surg*, 99(3), 324–335.

Nilsen, P. (2015). Making sense of implementation theories, models and frameworks. *Implement Sci*, 10(1), 53.

O'Mahony, D., O'Sullivan, D., Byrne, S., O'Connor, M.N., Ryan, C., & Gallagher, P. (2015). STOPP/START criteria for potentially inappropriate prescribing in older people: version 2. *Age Ageing*, 44(2), 213–218.

Palinkas, L.A., et al. (2015). Measuring sustainment of prevention programs and initiatives: a study protocol. *Implement Sci*, 11(1), 95.

Pearson, A., Jordan, Z., & Munn, Z. (2012). Translational science and evidence-based healthcare: a clarification and reconceptualization of how knowledge is generated and used in healthcare. *Nurs Res Pract*, 2012, 792519. doi:10.1155/2012/792519

Perla, R.J., Provost, L.P., & Parry, G.J. (2013). Seven propositions of the science of improvement: exploring foundations. *Qual Manag Healthcare*, 22(3), 170–186.

Powell, B.J., et al. (2015). A refined compilation of implementation strategies: results from the Expert Recommendations for Implementing Change (ERIC) project. *Implement Sci*, 10(1), 21.

Powell, B.J., et al. (2017). Methods to improve the selection and tailoring of implementation strategies. *J Behav Health Serv Res*, 44(2), 177–194.

Proctor, E., et al. (2011). Outcomes for implementation research: conceptual distinctions, measurement challenges, and research agenda. *Adm Policy Ment Health*, 38, 65–76. doi: 10.1007/s10488-010-0319-7

Proctor, E.K., Powell, B.J., & McMillen, J.C. (2013). Implementation strategies: recommendations for specifying and reporting. *Implement Sci*, 8, 139.

Public Health England. (2017). *English Surveillance Programme for Antimicrobial Utilisation and Resistance (ESPAUR) Report 2017.* London: Public Health England.

Reason, J. (2000). Human error: models and management. *BMJ*, 320(7237), 768–770.

Reason, J. (2016). *Managing the Risks of Organizational Accidents.* Routledge.

Reason, J., Hollnagel, E., & Paries, J. (2006). Revisiting the Swiss cheese model of accidents. *J Clin Eng*, 27, 110–115.

Russ, S., et al. (2015a). Measuring variation in use of the WHO surgical safety checklist in the operating room: a multicenter prospective cross-sectional study. *J Am Coll Surg*, 220(1), 1–11, e4.

Russ, S.J., et al. (2015b). A qualitative evaluation of the barriers and facilitators toward implementation of the WHO surgical safety checklist across hospitals in England: lessons from the 'Surgical Checklist Implementation Project'. *Ann Surg*, 261(1), 81–91.

Tabak, R.G., Khoong, E.C., Chambers, D.A., & Brownson, R.C. (2012). Bridging research and practice: models for dissemination and implementation research. *Am J Prev Med*, 43(3), 337–350.

Taylor–Adams, S. & Vincent, C. (2004). Systems analysis of clinical incidents: the London protocol. *Clin Risk*, 10(6), 211–220.

Taylor, M.J., McNicholas, C., Nicolay, C., Darzi, A., Bell, D., & Reed, J.E. (2014). Systematic review of the application of quality improvement methodologies from the manufacturing industry to surgical healthcare. *BMJ Qual Saf*, 23(4), 290–298.

Urbach, D.R., Govindarajan, A., Saskin, R., Wilton, A.S., & Baxter, N.N. (2014). Introduction of surgical safety checklists in Ontario, Canada. *New Engl J Med*, 370(11), 1029–1038.

Varkey, P., Reller, M.K., & Resar, R.K. (2007). Basics of quality improvement in health care. *Mayo Clin Proc*, 82(6), 735–739.

Vincent, C. (2010). How to improve patient safety in surgery. *J Health Serv Res Policy*, 15(1 suppl), 40–43.

Vincent, C.A., Neale, G., & Woloshynowych, M. (2001). Adverse events in British hospitals: preliminary retrospective record review. *BMJ*, 322, 517–519.

Wahid, A., Moppett, S.H., & Moppett, I.K. (2016). Research quality of quality accounts: transparency of public reporting of never events in England. A semi-quantitative and qualitative review. *J R Soc Med*, 109(5), 190–199.

Weiner, B.J., et al. (2017). Psychometric assessment of three newly developed implementation outcome measures. *Implement Sci*, 12(1), 108.

Wooton, D. (2006). *Bad Medicine: Doctors Doing Harm Since Hippocrates*. Oxford: Oxford University Press.

World Health Organization. (2009). *Patient Safety Curriculum Guide for Medical Schools. Topic 3: Understanding Systems and the Impact of Complexity on Patient Care*. Geneva: World Health Organization. Available at: http://www.who.int/patientsafety/education/curriculum/download/en/

13
Health services for health promotion and disease prevention

Jenifer Smith and James Mapstone

13.1 Introduction

The World Health Organization identified 'health' as a 'state of complete physical, mental, and social wellbeing, and not merely the absence of disease or infirmity' (Leonardi, 2018). Consistent with this definition, the 'right to health' does not just depend on 'medical service and medical attention in the event of sickness' but also requires 'the prevention, treatment and control of epidemic, endemic, occupational and other diseases' (Office of the High Commissioner for Human Rights, 1976). In recent decades, advances in health technology have greatly increased the effectiveness of health services for the treatment of disease, including cancer and cardiovascular diseases as the major causes of mortality; but medical care forms only one component of improving the health of the population. Health services can make important contributions to broader public health efforts to prevent disease and promote health.

During the nineteenth century, disease prevention efforts mainly focused on the control of infectious disease. Poor sanitation was associated with the spread of cholera through the work of John Snow; Semmelweis discovered that hospital-acquired post-partum infection could be prevented through improved hand hygiene; Lister developed antiseptic techniques to prevent surgically acquired infections. During the twentieth century, development of epidemiological methods facilitated recognition of the importance of environmental and social factors such as clean air, housing, and wealth in determining the health of a population. This was accompanied by growing recognition of the importance of social deprivation over the life course in determining health status and in generating inequalities in health. Dahlgren and Whitehead (1991) emphasized the importance of community-level and environmental influences, and their relationship to individual behaviours and health status. In the later part of the twentieth century, academic writers like McKeown (1979) showed that medical care had made only limited contributions to historical reductions in mortality and the decline of diseases like tuberculosis.

The Canadian Minister of National Health and Welfare, Marc Lalonde, is widely credited with prompting a conceptual shift by distinguishing the policy objective of an effective healthcare system from the prevention of health problems and the

Jenifer Smith and James Mapstone, *Health services for health promotion and disease prevention* In: *Healthcare Public Health*. Edited by: Martin Gulliford and Edmund Jessop, Oxford University Press (2020). © Oxford University Press. DOI: 10.1093/oso/9780198837206.003.0013.

Table 13.1 Levels of prevention intervention

Level	Aim	Examples
Primary	To prevent the onset of disease	Immunization, seat-belt legislation
Secondary	To prevent the progression of disease after onset	Breast-cancer screening, antiplatelet drugs after stroke
Tertiary	To reduce the impact of an ongoing disease	Speech therapy following a stroke

promotion of good health. The 1974 Lalonde report ('A New Perspective on the Health of Canadians') emphasized the importance of risk factors for disease (including alcohol, tobacco, diet, and exercise) which are under individual control but are also highly dependent on environmental and community-level influences. It follows that to improve the health of a population, it is necessary to intervene at personal and societal levels across a wide range of disciplines and agencies. In the Alma Ata Declaration, the World Health Organization (1978) promoted universal access to primary healthcare as a strategy for achieving better population health: the concept of primary healthcare was not limited to the delivery of medical services but also included health education to improve health literacy, ensuring access to a healthy diet and safe water, immunization against important diseases, and the prevention and control of locally endemic diseases. These pioneering documents brought a new focus to the question of how health services can contribute to the prevention of disease and improvements in health, but health services have generally been slow to embrace their responsibilities in this regard, because the short-term outcomes of urgent medical treatment will often be more tangible than the long-term outcomes of preventive medical interventions. The remainder of this chapter concentrates on those aspects which can be directed through health services by one or more of leadership, advocacy, partnership, or direct service provision.

13.2 Strategies for prevention

13.2.1 Levels of prevention

Disease prevention is often categorized into levels of primary, secondary, and tertiary prevention (Table 13.1), but these labels are not always helpful. Primary prevention is usually defined as preventing the onset of a disease and is often focused on reducing or eliminating risk factors. Smoking cessation before an individual has a smoking-related disease is an example of primary prevention. Primary prevention may focus on enhancing resilience, as when walking in nature may enhance resilience to mental illness. Secondary prevention is defined as identifying the disease in an early or asymptomatic phase and intervening to prevent progression. Cancer screening programmes or the detection and treatment of early and uncomplicated type II diabetes fall into this category. Tertiary prevention occurs after diagnosis of a disease and is focused on reducing its impact. This includes rehabilitation as well as treating established complications of the disease.

The idea of levels for prevention intervention is widely used in the scientific literature, as well as in policy documents, with the implication that the categories are mutually exclusive and easily distinguished. However, this is not always the case. Smoking cessation in the absence of disease can be classified as primary prevention, but smoking cessation is even more important after the onset of disease and is then classified as secondary prevention. This confusion may be compounded by differing views on what constitutes a disease. Elevated blood pressure is a risk factor for cardiovascular disease, but a diagnosis of 'hypertension' might appear to indicate the presence of a cardiovascular abnormality that might have been prevented. It is not clear whether treating high blood pressure represents a strategy for primary prevention of cardiovascular disease, or whether this is secondary prevention of an existing cardiovascular abnormality. Patients with high blood pressure may have subclinical atheromatous disease, and the approach to prevention should not just depend on whether individuals have already had clinically apparent cardiovascular events. Similarly, obesity is a risk factor, but patients with body mass index values of greater than 40 kg/m^2 may be disabled by their obesity and require weight reduction as a rehabilitation intervention. Depending on whether obesity is defined as a risk factor or a disease, intervention might be defined as a primary, secondary, or tertiary prevention.

There is also a difficulty that levels of prevention may be confused with levels of care and the setting in which prevention interventions are delivered, with primary prevention being the focus in the community, leaving hospital and specialist care to focus on secondary and tertiary prevention. The danger of this misunderstanding is that it can be a barrier to appreciating the importance of prevention, and ensuring its appropriate delivery, throughout the care pathway. For these reasons, the modern approach to the design, delivery, and evaluation of a prevention programme does not distinguish these levels of prevention.

13.2.2 Population-wide and high-risk approaches

In his writing on the 'Strategy of Preventive Medicine', the British epidemiologist Geoffrey Rose (1992) introduced the concept that public health interventions may either be directed at entire populations or targeted at individuals who are at high risk. Risk factors are often distributed on a continuous scale. Systolic blood pressure (SBP) shows a slightly skewed distribution, with a mean of about 120 mm Hg and standard deviation of about 18 mm Hg in many populations. The high-risk strategy for intervention is to identify individuals with the highest blood pressures and engage them in lifestyle interventions or blood pressure treatment. Individuals with the highest blood pressure values are an appropriate group for targeted intervention because they have the highest relative and absolute risks of cardiovascular events, including myocardial infarctions and strokes. A high-risk approach is consistent with the clinical approach to diagnosis and management of health conditions, and those at high risk may be particularly motivated to improve their health. The targeted approach may also allow cost-effective use of resources, which will be allocated where benefits are greatest. However, the high-risk approach also has disadvantages. It may be difficult to dichotomize the continuous blood pressure distribution. The threshold for diagnosis of hypertension has been revised over time from 160/95 mm Hg to 140/90 mm Hg; and in some groups, such as people with diabetes, a lower threshold may be preferred. The high-risk approach has the effect of medicalizing disease prevention. This is particularly relevant for lifestyle change interventions aimed at individuals, which may have limited effect if the wider social and environmental context remains unchanged.

Rose (1992) pointed out the 'prevention paradox': a majority of cardiovascular events are expected to arise in individuals who have normal or only mildly elevated risk-factor values, while only a minority occur in those at high risk. This is because a much larger proportion of the population is exposed in these lower-risk categories. A high-risk strategy will not impact on the risks of this wider group. A population-wide prevention strategy aims to reduce the population mean risk-factor value; this will reduce risk throughout the risk-factor distribution. This will also reduce the number of individuals at high risk because, as Rose pointed out, the number of deviant individuals with values above a given cut-off point depends on the population mean value (Rose & Day, 1990).

The North Karelia Cardiovascular Prevention Project in Finland provides an example of a population-wide intervention strategy (Puska et al., 1979). This project aimed at reducing the very high mortality rates from ischaemic heart disease in North Karelia by reducing the prevalence of its major risk factors—particularly smoking, high blood pressure, and serum total cholesterol—in the general population. The intervention strategy included campaigns in the mass media; interventions at schools, community organizations, and workplaces; training of GPs and nurses in polyclinics to undertake health and lifestyle checks; and encouraging food manufacturers to reduce the fat content of foods. The population-wide approach enables people to live in a healthier environment, thereby facilitating healthier behaviours. However, the resources for prevention are allocated to all individuals, including those at low as well as high risk, and the former group may have limited motivation to change their behaviour.

Disease prevention strategies often represent complex interventions with several components, and may combine both population-wide and high-risk approaches at different stages of the disease pathway. Health services sometimes deploy a population-wide approach, as in screening and immunization, but may often have a role in identifying and intervening with those at high risk, while population-wide approaches are delivered through wider health improvement strategies that target determinants of health.

The Diabetes Prevention Programme in England provides an example of a programme that employs an exclusively high-risk strategy. Individuals at high risk of Type 2 diabetes need to be identified by a physiological metric suitable for use at scale and measurable by non-invasive and widely acceptable means. Neither fasting blood glucose measurements nor glucose tolerance tests, which form the basis of the WHO definition of diabetes, are suitable. In 2011, the WHO concluded that the convenience of HbA1c measurement outweighed the difficulty of quality assuring its use, and determined that the threshold for a diagnosis of diabetes should be 48 mmol/mol (6.5%). In England, participants with HbA1c values of 42–47 mmol/mol (6.00–6.49%) are classified as having non-diabetic hyperglycaemia and are eligible for the Diabetes Prevention Programme (NHS England, 2016). Different criteria are used in other countries. An alternative approach is to select individuals as high risk based on data from electronic health records for family history, body mass index, age, ethnicity, and use of corticosteroids (Griffin et al., 2001).

The distinction of population-wide and high-risk approaches can also be applied to the prevention of infectious diseases. The English seasonal influenza programme (Box 13.1) provides an example of a programme that uses a targeted approach. However, there are elements that are population-wide, with the aim of achieving population impact using a number of different settings to deliver the overall aim, drawing on international evidence, with continuous review and development. An annual review of the influenza vaccination programme informs priorities for the year ahead and influences public and professional communications from the Chief Medical Officer. In the 2018/2019 influenza season, the vaccination programme utilized community, primary care, and secondary care settings to maximize the uptake of the seasonal flu vaccine. Vaccine uptake is reported monthly throughout the season, with weekly reporting from a subset of general practices.

13.2.3 Upstream and downstream intervention: proximal and distal causes

Public health makes a distinction between upstream and downstream intervention. Downstream prevention interventions are targeted at proximal or immediate causes of health problems but may fail to address root causes. Bariatric surgery is an example of a downstream intervention: it is effective at causing obese individuals to lose weight and reduces their risk of complications, but deployment of the procedure is unlikely to impact on the obesity epidemic because it does not address the causes of obesity. Upstream interventions aim to intervene on distal or underlying social and economic determinants of health in order to enable people to achieve their full health potential. The 'sugar tax', which aims to reduce consumption of excessive amounts of sugars in soft drinks, is an example of an upstream intervention (Colchero et al., 2016). Adams et al. (2016) discussed disease prevention interventions in terms of their level of individual agency. 'High-agency' interventions require a high level of individual

Box 13.1 Influenza vaccination programme

All pre-school children aged 2 to 3 years: included in a programme delivered by general practices. The parents of all children registered by the practice receive an invitation for their child to receive vaccinations.

All children aged 4 to 9 years: included in a school-based programme. This achieves higher uptake than the pre-school component because response to an invitation is not required. The aim of influenza vaccination in children is to prevent morbidity and mortality from influenza in individuals and also to reduce influenza transmission in the community.

People with defined serious medical conditions: offered influenza vaccination between the ages of 6 months and 65 years. The programme is delivered by general practices, with support by community pharmacies, and sometimes in specific secondary care settings such as renal dialysis units. The aim of this programme, and the one for those over 65 years of age, is to prevent morbidity and mortality in individuals.

People aged 65 years and over: offered influenza vaccination by their general practices, supported by community pharmacies. This programme has the highest uptake of all the component influenza vaccination programmes.

All pregnant women: offered influenza vaccination with the aim of reducing morbidity and mortality in pregnant women, and protecting the foetus and newborn in the first few months of life. This is delivered by general practices, supported by community pharmacies, and also by local maternity services in the community and hospital settings.

Other groups: there are components of the programme for carers, and health and social care workers. Some employers also invest in flu vaccination as part of their occupational programmes; and the vaccine is available, for a fee, from community pharmacies for people who wish to have it who fall outside these categories.

Source: data from Department of Health and Social Care (2019). 'The national flu immunisation programme 2018/19'. London: Department of Health and Social Care. Available at: https://assets.publishing.service.gov.uk/government/uploads/system/uploads/attachment_data/file/694779/Annual_national_flu_programme_2018-2019.pdf

engagement, effort, and investment of resources as, for example, in individual diet and physical exercise counselling. 'Low-agency' interventions, such as the fortification of flour with folic acid or fluoridation of the water supply, require little engagement from individuals, but may be criticized for being apparently paternalistic and possibly infringing individual autonomy. The World Health Organization (2002) recommends that it is generally more effective to give priority to population-wide interventions that focus on primary prevention through intervention on distal rather than proximal risks to health.

13.3 Prevention programmes

There are three overlapping and equally important phases to the delivery of a prevention programme that will have an impact at a population level: design, implementation, and improvement and evaluation. Delivering prevention programmes requires multidisciplinary expertise because few people have all the skills necessary to deliver all phases. It is important to the success of a programme that team roles are clearly defined and consistent with individuals' skills. It is also important to engage with stakeholders, including people who will be delivering the programme, as well as service users and a wider public. Without effective engagement and involvement, a programme is likely to fail to meet its objectives.

A prevention programme should start with an overall aim, but this should be accompanied by intermediate goals that may appear more tangible and may help to inspire contributors to help deliver the programme. Working with key stakeholders can help to develop the specification of overarching aims and intermediate goals. A public health specialist may have a passion to reduce smoking prevalence in the community by delivering brief interventions in hospital settings, but an intermediate goal of reducing the need for secondary care services in winter may increase engagement of hospital-based staff whose assistance is needed.

13.3.1 Priorities for prevention

Having established that a health service programme should include disease prevention interventions, the next question to address is what objectives should be included. Needs assessment and resource prioritization will generally be required, as outlined in other chapters, in order to refine the programme's intended purpose of improving the health of the population through actions within the remit of the healthcare sector. The burden of illness in a population is usually described in terms of mortality and morbidity, so an assessment of how prevention could make an impact on the major causes is appropriate. Many causes of mortality are also at the root of much ill health within a population, but the burden of disease in a population may include some disabling conditions with comparatively low mortality rates. The Global Burden of Disease Study employs the disability adjusted life year (DALY) as a metric that combines both mortality and disability, and this has been important in drawing attention to the large burden of illness from common mental health disorders. In the study results for 2017, the risk factors that accounted for the largest global share of DALYs were high SBP, smoking, high body mass index and elevated plasma glucose, and short gestation for birthweight (Stanaway et al., 2018). In analyses for the UK in 2013, ischaemic heart disease accounted for the greatest number of life years lost, but low back and neck pain accounted for most DALYs. The risk factors accounting for the greatest burden of DALYs were suboptimal diet and tobacco smoking (Newton et al., 2015).

13.3.2 Evidence of effectiveness and cost effectiveness

The design of a programme should be informed by existing evidence concerning the effectiveness of interventions. This should draw on systematic reviews and meta-analyses of well-conducted randomized controlled trials. Box 13.2 provides an example of a

---

Box 13.2 Use of evidence in the design of a diabetes prevention programme

Needs assessment

Type 2 diabetes is one of the fastest growing causes of ill health in many countries worldwide, fuelled by the rapidly increasing prevalence of obesity. In England, up to six per cent of the population currently have diabetes. The increase in prevalence has been accompanied by a growing burden of illness from complications including amputations, renal failure, cardiovascular diseases, and blindness. The rapid increase in obesity in children and young adults has been accompanied by increasing numbers of cases of diabetes in young people (Abbasi et al., 2016). People of Indian subcontinent or Black African and Caribbean origins are up to six times more likely to develop Type 2 diabetes, and do so at younger ages and at lower body mass index values than people of European origins.

Physical inactivity is an independent risk factor for diabetes, and while increasing activity is likely to be an element of a campaign to reduce obesity, it will be an important element of a programme to reduce diabetes. A national obesity prevention strategy may contribute to the prevention of Type 2 diabetes and other diseases, but alone is insufficient and needs to be supplemented by a behavioural intervention targeted at those at high risk of developing diabetes.

Evidence of effectiveness

The effectiveness of diabetes prevention interventions was evaluated in a meta-analysis of 17 randomized controlled trials that included participants with impaired glucose tolerance. The meta-analysis found that lifestyle interventions were associated with a relative risk of diabetes of 0.51 (95% confidence interval 0.44 to 0.60); one case of diabetes was estimated to be prevented for each 6.4 (95% confidence interval 5.0 to 8.4) participants receiving lifestyle advice (Gillies et al., 2007).

This review provided strong evidence that lifestyle advice of increased physical activity, healthy diet, and weight reduction could be effective at reducing the incidence of Type 2 diabetes in people with impaired glucose tolerance as a marker of high risk.

In an updated systematic review, Ashra et al. (2015) found that intensive group-based behavioural interventions oriented towards achieving a healthy weight, eating a healthy diet, and undertaking recommended levels of daily activity could prevent or delay the onset of Type 2 diabetes in people with non-diabetic hyperglycaemia.

diabetes prevention intervention. Brief interventions by doctors and nurses have been found to be effective in reducing excessive alcohol intake (Kaner et al., 2007) or promoting physical activity (Orrow et al., 2012), but effects are generally small or absent for obesity and body-weight advice (Booth et al., 2014) and cardiovascular risk management (Alageel et al., 2017). Effectiveness estimates can be incorporated into health economic modelling studies that predict the long-term costs and outcomes of preventive intervention programmes. These may be employed to justify the use of resources in terms of the return on investment (ROI), defined as the expected value generated by an investment in relation to the resources required. Other types of evidence are also needed in order to understand the potential uptake, reach, and acceptability of an intervention programme, and these may be provided by drawing on previous experience in other places, including non-randomized evaluations and grey literature. Advice from experts in the field, and engagement with patients and the public, may contribute important insights into how to implement the programme that is being planned.

13.3.3 Behaviour change techniques

Prevention interventions often promote changes in behaviour from healthcare providers, patients, service users, and members of the public. Consequently, it is important to draw on behavioural science expertise to aid in the design and implementation of a prevention programme. This will focus on the theoretical basis for the intervention and the nature of the active behaviour change ingredients that should be incorporated into an effective intervention. Health psychologists and other experts in behaviour change have been active in developing structured tools that can inform the development and delivery of behaviour change interventions (Atkins et al., 2017; Michie et al., 2014). There is a substantial body of knowledge available concerning which behaviour change tools are likely to be effective and which ones are unlikely to work in a given context. It is important to ensure that preventive healthcare interventions are informed by these behavioural insights in order to ensure achievable standards of efficacy in behaviour change. It is also important that the healthcare workforce develops more sophisticated skills in behaviour change techniques (Keyworth et al., 2019) because we know that traditional methods, such as simply communicating information about risks, are not effective at changing peoples' behaviours (Marteau, 2018). Many prevention interventions have either failed to consider, or have failed to report on, the intended theoretical mechanisms of effect and the active behaviour change ingredients of their interventions. Unsurprisingly, many of these poorly designed interventions were found to be ineffective (Alageel et al., 2017; Dalgetty et al., 2019).

13.3.4 Logic models

Prevention interventions can be structured with a logic model that identifies the overall aim and shows the processes through which the planned project or programme

---

Box 13.3 Developing a logic model for a smoking cessation brief intervention

---

- Make realistic assumptions of how many people would receive the intervention (e.g. 80% of clinic attenders). Be clear on the population targeted for intervention.
- Use local information, where possible, of the proportion of people receiving the intervention who will be smokers. This will vary by clinic but assume 40% for this example.
- Use evidence from randomized trials about the effectiveness of a brief intervention in an outpatient setting. For example, the number needed to receive a brief intervention to create an additional non-smoker at six months is of the order of 50 (Stead et al., 2012).
- Estimate the number of myocardial infarcts and strokes prevented by the programme, making a set of reasonable assumptions concerning the reduction in risk of both from someone giving up smoking compared to continuing.

---

will lead to expected outcomes. A logic model is a statement, often represented as an infographic, that shows how an intervention strategy is intended to achieve its objectives (Public Health England, 2018). The logic model will summarize the programme inputs in terms of resources, the implementation activities as outputs, the context as a moderating factor, and the outcomes of the programme in terms of its health impacts. It brings together the way the effectiveness of the individual interventions feeds through to the ultimate aim (Public Health England, 2018). Box 13.3 considers how a brief intervention on smoking, in secondary care outpatient clinics, may lead to reduced winter admissions. If the logic model suggests the overall aim is not achievable, it will be necessary to reconsider the proposed intervention or add in additional interventions. Finally, a clear programme or project plan is required for agreement between all partners. This must include clear deliverables, timescales, resources, and governance.

13.3.5 Programme implementation

Implementation requires a different set of skills to designing the programme. While the design of a programme often benefits greatly from the input of individuals with implementation expertise, it does not follow that implementation is best led by the same individuals that were responsible for programme design. In the implementation phase, the design team has a role in ensuring fidelity to the overall aim and rationale, and to help in revising the logic model to take account of planned changes to the programme. The concept of fidelity refers to the degree to which programmes are implemented as intended by developers (Carroll et al., 2007). There is increasing interest in adaptive implementation, which allows for planned enhancements to the intervention strategy at sites where initial results suggest that objectives may not be being achieved (Kilbourne et al., 2014).

Implementation is rarely easy and often requires resilience, tenacity, and a sense of humour. People delivering the programme, and those it is aimed at, need to be inspired and encouraged to be part of this new programme. Identifying a 'champion' for the programme at each site is one strategy for achieving this (Soo et al., 2009). Robust management and governance structures are essential so that problems arising from the implementation are identified early and rectified.

In the Diabetes Prevention Programme in England, the strategy for intervention is specified in accordance with a national framework. It has the core goals of promoting weight loss, improving diet, and increasing physical activity levels, and with the incorporation of behaviour change techniques in intervention delivery. The intervention is delivered to groups of 15 to 20 participants during a minimum of 13 sessions over a period of nine months (Penn et al., 2018). A national commissioning model was adopted to take advantage of the purchasing power this enables, together with maintaining fidelity to a core specification. In order to generate local ownership and enable connection to local communities and their assets, a framework of providers capable of delivering on a national scale was established, with local competitive tendering exercises for local health systems to select their preferred provider. In this model, local health systems are responsible for generating referrals into the service and working with their chosen provider to ensure service delivery reflects the needs of the local population. In particular, this requires addressing ethnic and socioeconomic diversity to avoid introducing inequalities in outcome.

13.3.6 Evaluation

Evaluation of the prevention programme needs to be an integral part of the programme from the design phase. Evaluation by a team that is independent of programme management is often desirable. The evaluation team will require expertise in health measurement, statistical analysis, health economic evaluation, and qualitative research, among other areas. The primary and secondary health and health economic outcome measures on which the success of the programme will be judged should be clearly prespecified, with reliable and valid data-collection procedures being established and tested.

The evaluation design should include a comparator that permits estimation of the counterfactual (i.e. the outcome that might have occurred in the absence of a prevention programme). Randomized designs, including cluster randomized trials, provide rigorous evaluation but are not always feasible or politically acceptable. There is growing interest in the step-wedge design, which allows all sites to engage in an intervention but in a randomized sequence (Hemming et al., 2015). Non-randomized interrupted time series and difference-in-difference designs may be employed if randomization is not feasible (Wing et al., 2018). These elements of the evaluation will provide evidence for the effectiveness and cost effectiveness of an intervention programme.

Process evaluation is also required (Moore et al., 2015) and typically uses mixed methods to gain insights into the implementation of the planned programme, including intervention fidelity, uptake, and adaptations; the mechanisms through which the programme had effect; and any contextual factors that impacted on the effectiveness of the programme.

13.4 Conclusions

Population ageing is being accompanied by increasing multiple morbidity, with a consequent burden on health services. Promoting healthy ageing and preventing the onset of long-term conditions is now a high priority. This chapter has provided an overview of the approaches and methods through which health services can achieve disease prevention objectives. It is essential that the actions of health services are co-ordinated with broader public health efforts to improve population health and reduce inequalities through intervention on determinants of health.

References

Abbasi, A., Juszczyk, D., van Jaarsveld, C.H.M., & Gulliford, M.C. (2016). Body-mass index and incidence of type 1 and type 2 diabetes in children and young adults in the UK: an observational cohort study. *Lancet*, 388, 16.

Adams, J., Mytton, O., White, M., & Monsivais, P. (2016). Why are some population interventions for diet and obesity more equitable and effective than others? The role of individual agency. *PLoS Med*, 13(4), e1001990. doi: 10.1371/journal.pmed.1001990

Alageel, S., Gulliford, M.C., McDermott, L., & Wright, A.J. (2017). Multiple health behaviour change interventions for primary prevention of cardiovascular disease in primary care: systematic review and meta-analysis. *BMJ Open*, 7, e015375.

Ashra, N.B., et al. (2015). *A systematic review and metaanalysis assessing the effectiveness of pragmatic lifestyle interventions for the prevention of type 2 diabetes mellitus in routine practice*. London: Public Health England.

Atkins, L., et al. (2017). A guide to using the Theoretical Domains Framework of behaviour change to investigate implementation problems. *Implement Sci*, 12, 77.

Booth, H.P., Prevost, A.T., Wright, A.J., & Gulliford, M.C. (2014). Effectiveness of behavioral weight loss interventions delivered in a primary care setting: a systematic review and meta-analysis. *Fam Pract*, 31(6), 643–653.

Carroll, C., Patterson, M., Wood, S., Booth, A., Rick, J., & Balain, S. (2007). A conceptual framework for implementation fidelity. *Implement Sci*, 2, 40.

Colchero, M.A., Popkin, B.M., Rivera, J.A., & Ng, S.W. (2016). Beverage purchases from stores in Mexico under the excise tax on sugar sweetened beverages: observational study. *BMJ*, 352, h6704.

Dahlgren, G. & Whitehead, M. (1991). *Policies and Strategies to Promote Social Equity in Health*. Stockholm, Sweden: Institute for Futures Studies. Available at: https://core.ac.uk/download/pdf/6472456.pdf [accessed 17 July 2019].

Dalgetty, R., Miller, C.B., & Dombrowski, S.U. (2019). Examining the theory-effectiveness hypothesis: a systematic review of systematic reviews. *Br J Health Psychol*, 24, 334–356.

Department of Health and Social Care. (2019). *The National Flu Immunisation Programme 2018/19*. London: Department of Health and Social Care. Available at: https://assets.publishing.service.gov.uk/government/uploads/system/uploads/attachment_data/file/694779/Annual_national_flu_programme_2018-2019.pdf [accessed 17 July 2019].

Gillies, C.L., et al. (2007). Pharmacological and lifestyle interventions to prevent or delay type 2 diabetes in people with impaired glucose tolerance: systematic review and meta-analysis. *BMJ*, 334, 299.

Griffin, S.J., Little, P.S., Hales, C.N., Kinmonth, A.L., & Wareham, N.J. (2001). Diabetes risk score: towards earlier detection of type 2 diabetes in general practice. *Diabetes Metab Res Rev*, 16, 164–171.

Hemming, K., Haines, T.P., Chilton, P.J., Girling, A.J., & Lilford, R.J. (2015). The stepped wedge cluster randomised trial: rationale, design, analysis, and reporting. *BMJ*, 350, h391.

Kaner, E.F., et al. (2007). Effectiveness of brief alcohol interventions in primary care populations. *Cochrane Database Syst Rev*, Cd004148.

Keyworth, C., Epton, T., Goldthorpe, J., Calam, R., & Armitage, C.J. (2019) 'It's difficult, I think it's complicated': health care professionals' barriers and enablers to providing opportunistic behaviour change interventions during routine medical consultations. *Br J Health Psychol*, 24(3), 571–592.

Kilbourne, A.M., et al. (2014). Protocol: Adaptive Implementation of Effective Programs Trial (ADEPT): cluster randomized SMART trial comparing a standard versus enhanced implementation strategy to improve outcomes of a mood disorders program. *Implement Sci*, 9, 132.

Lalonde, M. (1974). *A New Perspective on the Health of Canadians*. Ottawa, ON: Minister of Supply and Services Canada. Available at: http://www.phac-aspc.gc.ca/ph-sp/pdf/perspect-eng.pdf [accessed 17 July 2019].

Leonardi, F. (2018). The definition of health: towards new perspectives. *Int J Health Serv*, 48, 735–748.

Marteau, T.M. (2018). Changing minds about changing behaviour. *Lancet*, 391, 116–117.

McKeown, T. (1979). *The Role of Medicine*. Oxford: Blackwell.

Michie, S., Atkins, L., & West, R. (2014). *The Behaviour Change Wheel—A Guide to Designing Interventions*. Great Britain: Silverback Publishing.

Moore, G.F., et al. (2015). Process evaluation of complex interventions: Medical Research Council guidance. *BMJ*, 350, h1258.

Newton, J.N., et al. (2015). Changes in health in England, with analysis by English regions and areas of deprivation, 1990–2013: a systematic analysis for the Global Burden of Disease Study 2013. *Lancet*, 386, 2257–2274.

NHS England. (2016). *NHS Diabetes Prevention Programme and Weight Management Services: Eligibility Criteria*. London: NHS England. Available at: https://www.england.nhs.uk/wp-content/uploads/2016/07/dpp-wm-service.pdf [accessed 17 July 2019].

Office of the High Commissioner for Human Rights. (1976). International Covenant on Economic, Social and Cultural Rights. Geneva: Office of the High Commissioner for Human Rights. Available at: https://www.ohchr.org/en/professionalinterest/pages/cescr.aspx [accessed 17 July 2019].

Orrow, G., Kinmonth, A.-L., Sanderson, S., & Sutton, S. (2012). Effectiveness of physical activity promotion based in primary care: systematic review and meta-analysis of randomised controlled trials. *BMJ*, 344, e1389.

Penn, L., et al. (2018). NHS Diabetes Prevention Programme in England: formative evaluation of the programme in early phase implementation. *BMJ Open*, 8, e019467.

Public Health England. (2018). *Introduction to Logic Models*. London: Public Health England. Available at: https://www.gov.uk/government/publications/evaluation-in-health-and-well-being-overview/introduction-to-logic-models [accessed 17 July 2019].

Puska, P., et al. (1979). Changes in coronary risk factors during comprehensive five-year community programme to control cardiovascular diseases (North Karelia project). *BMJ*, 2, 1173–1178.

Rose, G. (1992). *The Strategy of Preventive Medicine*. Oxford: Oxford University Press.

Rose, G. & Day, S. (1990). The population mean predicts the number of deviant individuals [see comment]. *BMJ*, 301, 1031–1034.

Stanaway, J.D., et al. (2018). Global, regional, and national comparative risk assessment of 84 behavioural, environmental and occupational, and metabolic risks or clusters of risks for 195 countries and territories, 1990–2017: a systematic analysis for the Global Burden of Disease Study 2017. *Lancet*, 392, 1923–1994.

Stead, L.F., Perera, R., Bullen, C., Mant, D., & Lancaster, T. (2012) Nicotine replacement therapy for smoking cessation. *Cochrane Database Syst Rev*, CD000146.

Soo, S., Berta, W., & Baker, G.R. (2009). Role of champions in the implementation of patient safety practice change. *Healthc Q*, 12, 123–128.

Wing, C., Simon, K., & Bello–Gomez, R.A. (2018). Designing difference in difference studies: best practices for public health policy research. *Annu Rev Public Health*, 39(1), 453–469.

World Health Organization. (1978). Declaration of Alma-Ata. *WHO Chron*, 32, 428–430.

World Health Organization. (2002). *The World Health Report 2002—Reducing Risks, Promoting Healthy Life*. Geneva: World Health Organization.

14

Population screening

Allison Streetly and Nehmat Houssami

14.1 Introduction: definition of screening

Screening is a public health strategy for the prevention of disease through the early identification of health conditions, including diseases or predisease states, in individuals who presume themselves to be healthy. While the idea of population screening is attractive, and at first sight appears simple, the reality is that introducing formal screening programmes often raises ethical, conceptual, and practical challenges. It is important to understand why population screening differs in important respects from the investigation and treatment of symptomatic individuals who are already seeking healthcare intervention.

The term screening is often used loosely and inappropriately, but there are several clear definitions (Box 14.1). These definitions highlight different aspects of the screening process. The definition by the US Commission on Chronic Illness (1957) emphasizes that a screening test is not a diagnostic test and will usually need to be highly acceptable and low-cost for use in a population screening programme. McKeown (1976) draws attention to the ethical distinction from clinical practice, with screening tests being offered to individuals who believe themselves to be healthy. The UK National Screening Committee (2017) introduced the possible harms that may result from screening and the importance of balancing these against any possible benefits from early diagnosis and treatment. Raffle and Gray (2007) pointed out that possible benefits from screening may include reducing future risks of ill health. Benefit may also be possible if information is provided to assist decision making, even when eventual outcomes cannot be changed. For example, a pregnant woman who would not contemplate termination of pregnancy might choose to be screened for Down's syndrome, and if the baby is found to be affected, the parents and healthcare providers will have advance information; and for other parents, there may be choices concerning reproductive options.

In the UK, screening is implemented in the form of population-wide screening programmes comprising an organized strategy from invitation to be screened through to treatment. From a public health perspective, the systematic application of tests to patients in clinical settings does not represent 'screening', even though this term is often employed by clinicians. This is more appropriately referred to as 'opportunistic screening', 'testing', or 'case finding'. This approach to testing is very important in the clinical management of patients with long-term conditions. Clinical

Allison Streetly and Nehmat Houssami, *Population screening* In: *Healthcare Public Health*. Edited by: Martin Gulliford and Edmund Jessop, Oxford University Press (2020). © Oxford University Press. DOI: 10.1093/oso/9780198837206.003.0014.

Box 14.1 Definitions of screening

US Commission on Chronic Illness (1957): 'the presumptive identification of unrecognised disease or defect by the application of tests, examinations or other procedures that can be applied rapidly'.

McKeown (1976): 'medical investigation which does not arise from a patient's request for advice for a specific complaint'.

The UK National Screening Committee (2017): 'Screening is a public health service. The purpose of screening is to offer a test to members of a defined population who do not necessarily perceive that they are at risk of, or are already affected by, a disease or its complications. The test is to identify those individuals who are more likely to be helped than harmed by further tests or treatment to reduce the risk of disease or its complications.'

---

detection and management of atrial fibrillation may be employed to reduce stroke risk, even though population screening programmes for atrial fibrillation are not recommended at present (Orchard et al., 2018). In 2018, the US Preventive Services Task Force (2018a) found that while there was good evidence for clinical effectiveness of anticoagulation in atrial fibrillation, there was insufficient evidence that possible benefits of population-wide electrocardiographic screening might exceed the possible harms, including overdiagnosis and treatment of asymptomatic abnormalities.

14.2 Ethical questions in population screening

The decision to implement population screening raises important ethical questions, and it is important that these are considered at the earliest stage of screening programme development. In clinical practice, a person who believes they are unwell consults a doctor in the hope of obtaining benefit. This contrasts with population screening in which a decision is made at community-level to offer screening tests to individuals who may believe themselves to be healthy. From the community perspective, the allocation of resources to screening programmes must be justified in terms of the aggregate benefit that these programmes offer in relation to opportunity costs of alternative public health interventions that might not receive funding. The community perspective may also require that screening programmes achieve high population uptake in order to ensure that projected aggregate benefits are achieved and health inequalities are not increased through the introduction of screening.

The decision to implement a screening programme is generally motivated by the utilitarian idea of the 'greatest good for the greatest number' and is paternalistic in approach. This may cause tension with the ideal of individual autonomy, which requires that individuals have a choice of whether or not to engage with a screening invitation.

Screening programmes may result in significant harms to some individuals, conflicting with the principle of non-maleficence (Raffle & Gray, 2007). Treatment for abdominal aortic aneurysm, for example, is associated with appreciable mortality. Individuals must have the opportunity to value for themselves the impacts of possible benefits and harms from screening. People should participate in screening programmes on the basis of informed choice based on knowledge of what options the offer of a screening test will lead to. Marteau et al. (2001) defined informed choice as being 'based on relevant knowledge, consistent with decision-maker's values, and behaviourally implemented' (p. 100).

There have been considerable efforts in recent years to develop resources that can accompany screening invitations to provide information concerning possible benefits and harms, and inform individual decisions on whether or not to participate (Pace & Keating, 2014). This information is often provided at a sensitive time of life, for example, during pregnancy or just after the birth of a child. This may not be an optimal time to make decisions, and it is important to engage in education and communication with a wider public to ensure that the population is adequately informed and able to take decisions affecting their health.

Screening in the antenatal period raises ethical challenges on the valuation of outcomes when the test aims to identify risks of a disease in a foetus. For Down's syndrome screening, it is possible to estimate the cost per affected birth prevented, but it is ethically unacceptable to weigh this cost against the cost of treatment and care of affected individuals to justify its value. The possibility of making diagnoses before birth and giving parents informed choice over reproductive outcomes is regarded as the major positive benefit of this type of screening programme. Preconception screening may sometimes be a more appropriate time to offer carrier testing, with several countries introducing carrier screening for thalassaemia (Samavat & Modell, 2004). Despite this, preconception screening is not routinely established in many countries.

The increasing potential for genetic screening raises ethical issues. Genetic screening is generally most appropriate for single-gene disorders, such as cystic fibrosis and sickle cell disease. Newborn screening for sickle cell disease has now been introduced in America, Canada, in several European countries including the UK, and, slowly, in Africa (Streetly et al., 2018). More recently, screening has been proposed for familial hypercholesterolaemia (Wald et al., 2016). Proposals for whole-genome sequencing of all newborns, to allow identification of many rare genetic conditions and reduce diagnostic delay, have been rejected by expert bodies in the UK (The Nuffield Council on Bioethics, 2018). There is a risk that availability of genetic data could lead to discrimination on the basis of future health potential. Adequate genetic counselling is an essential prerequisite where such programmes are introduced.

14.3 Screening across the life course

In the UK, population screening programmes have mainly been developed for the antenatal and newborn period, as well as for selected cancers and cardiovascular

Table 14.1 Screening programmes in England

Condition	Test	Eligibility
Abdominal aortic aneurysm	Ultrasound scan	Men aged 65 years and over
Bowel cancer screening	Faecal occult blood test; fibre optic endoscopy	Men and women aged 60 to 74 years, every two years
Breast cancer	Mammographic screening	Women from 50 to 70 years inclusive; older women can self-refer
Cervical cancer	Cervical smear test	Women aged 25 to 49, every three years; women aged 50 to 64, every five years
Diabetic eye screening	Digital retinal photography	People with diabetes aged 12 years and over, annually
Antenatal and newborn screening	Haemoglobin disorders; infections; foetal anomalies; hearing; metabolic disorders; physical examination	Pregnant women and newborn infants

Source: data from Public Health England. (2019). *NHS Screening Timeline*. London: Public Health England.

disorders, as outlined in Table 14.1. There are no screening programmes for prostate cancer and lung cancer, even though these represent two of the most common cancers; nor do we have screening programmes for ischaemic heart disease and stroke. Section 14.4 discusses the criteria that are used to recommend the introduction of a population screening programme and explores why some important conditions do not meet these criteria.

14.4 Criteria for introducing a population screening programme

Wilson and Jungner suggested, in a report for the World Health Organization (Andermann et al., 2008), several criteria that could justify screening programmes. These criteria have been elaborated over time in order to acknowledge growing concern for the harms as well as possible benefits of screening, the importance of respecting individual autonomy and freedom of choice, and the potential impact of screening on health inequalities. In the UK, the National Screening Committee (2015) now employs the criteria shown in Box 14.2. The criteria broadly relate to the nature of the condition, the test to be used, the nature of interventions that might provide benefits, as well as criteria related to the screening programme and its implementation.

Box 14.2 Criteria for introducing a population screening programme

The condition

The condition should be an important health problem.

The epidemiology of the condition should be understood.

All the cost-effective primary prevention interventions should have been implemented.

The test

There should be a simple, safe, valid test.

The test values in the target population should be known and a suitable cut-off level agreed.

The test, from sample collection to delivery of results, should be acceptable.

There should be an agreed policy on investigation and choices for positive results (including genetic variants).

The intervention

There should be an effective intervention which leads to better outcomes than later detection and, where relevant, takes into account benefits to the wider family.

The screening programme

There should be evidence from high-quality randomized controlled trials that the screening programme is effective in reducing mortality or morbidity, or where the test relates to informed decision making (such as Down's syndrome screening), there must be evidence that the outcome is of value.

The complete screening programme is clinically, socially, and ethically acceptable.

The benefits gained from the screening programme should outweigh harms.

The opportunity cost of the screening programme should provide value for money.

Implementation criteria

Clinical management should be optimized before introducing of a screening programme.

Screening should be the most cost-effective intervention available.

Monitoring and quality assurance processes and standards should be part of the implementation plan.

Resources, including for information for all elements of the screening programme, should be available.

Adapted from United Kingdom National Screening Committee (2015). *Criteria for Appraising the Viability, Effectiveness and Appropriateness of a Screening Programme*. London: Department of Health and Social Care. Available at: https://www.gov.uk/government/publications/evidence-review-criteria-national-screening-programmes/criteria-for-appraising-the-viability-effectiveness-and-appropriateness-of-a-screening-programme

Conditions selected for screening should generally represent an important burden of disease either in terms of their high frequency or because of their high impact on affected individuals. It is also important that the natural history of disease, including progression from latent to clinically manifest stages, is well understood. Screening represents a form of secondary prevention intervention, and conditions that are amenable to effective primary prevention intervention will less often be suitable targets for screening programmes. Tests employed in screening programmes should generally be simple, safe, and highly acceptable to the target population. Any screening test should provide valid results, and this requires consensus on how to define abnormal results that require further investigation. These important properties of screening tests are discussed further in Section 14.5.

It should be noted that while these criteria may imply a binary choice of meeting the criteria or not, most existing national screening programmes broadly meet these criteria but may include criteria that are only partially satisfied. This is considered further in the section on cessation of screening programmes which, like their commencement, can be influenced by political decisions.

14.5 Screening test evaluation

Screening test validity is conventionally described in terms of sensitivity and specificity (Figure 14.1). Sensitivity is defined as the proportion of subjects with the condition of interest who are classified as true positives by the test. A sensitive test is one that detects a high proportion of affected cases. Specificity is defined as the proportion of disease-free subjects who are classified as true negatives by the test. A specific test is one that gives few positive results when the condition is absent. Sensitivity and specificity are often referred to as properties of a test, but they may also depend on patient characteristics and may vary in different groups of patients. The estimation of sensitivity and specificity also requires dichotomization of test results and disease risk, and this may not always be optimal from clinical and statistical perspectives.

When test results are reported on a continuous scale, the threshold or cut-point to define an abnormal result can be adjusted. Lowering the threshold will generally have the effect of increasing test sensitivity, allowing a higher proportion of cases to be identified as test positives, but this is at the price of reduced specificity, as more disease-free individuals test positive too. Conversely, increasing the threshold can result in increased specificity but sensitivity will be reduced. Global test performance is often reported in terms of the area under the receiver operating characteristic (ROC) curve (Figure 14.2). The ROC curve plots the relationship between the proportions of true positive results (sensitivity) and false positive results (1−specificity) for all possible test cut-points. There are several methods for determining the optimal cut-point: a well-known criterion is the greatest value for the Youden index calculated as sensitivity + specificity − 1.

In the context of screening programmes, the positive predictive value (PPV) of a test is of great importance (Figure 14.1). This is defined as the proportion of subjects with a positive test result who have the condition of interest. The predictive value of a test varies with the prevalence of a condition. In high-prevalence settings like hospitals, where tests may be developed, true positives will be frequent. However, in low-prevalence settings, among whole populations in the community, true positives will be infrequent, false positives more frequent, and the predictive value of the test low. Conditions that are sought by screening programmes, even if considered to be frequent conditions, commonly have a prevalence of less than 1% (typically <0.8% in population breast screening). When a condition is rare, individuals without the condition represent a high proportion of those undergoing the test. Consequently, false positive results will generally outnumber true positive results and the predictive value of a screening test will be low. Improving the specificity of a screening test is particularly important to minimize the harms associated with false positive results, including additional investigations and treatment as well as the anxiety accompanying a possible serious diagnosis.

Optimizing *specificity* becomes important for an effective and acceptable programme because the number of false positives will usually outweigh true positives. This significantly impacts on the costs and acceptability of such programmes. Using data from Australia's national population-based breast screening programme, BreastScreen Australia, from 823,364 women aged 50–74 years in 2015 and having repeat screening in the BreastScreen programme, 31,344 (3.8%) had a positive screen and were recalled for further assessment, resulting in the detection of 5,610 invasive or *in situ* cancers (0.7% of screens)—so the PPV was 18% and for each true positive (TP) screen there were 4.6 false positive (FP) screens (Australian Institute of Health and Welfare, 2017). The number needed to screen (NNS) to detect one invasive breast cancer decreases with increasing age group, reflecting the higher underlying cancer incidence and prevalence in older women (as well as relatively higher mammography sensitivity in older groups), as follows: NNS 270 (45–49 years), NNS 250 (50–54 years), NNS 217 (55–59 years), NNS 179 (60–64 years), and NNS 145 (65–69) years.

	Disease Present	Disease Absent	
Test result Positive	True Positive (TP)	False Positive (FP)	**Positive Predictive Value** = TP/(TP+FP)
Test result Negative	False Negative (FN)	True Negative (TN)	**Negative Predictive Value** = TN/(TN+FN)
	Sensitivity = TP/(TP+FN)	Specificity = TN/(TN+FP)	

Figure 14.1 Analysing screening test results.

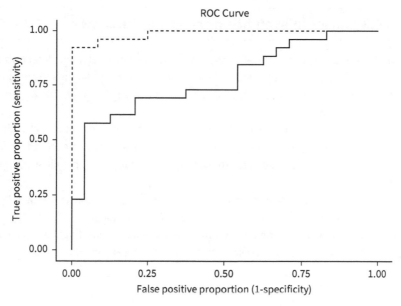

Figure 14.2 Examples of receiver operating characteristic (ROC) curves.

14.6 Screening programme effectiveness

A screening programme does not only rely on having a good screening test. The justification for screening lies in the potentially better health outcomes for people with screen-detected disease, as compared to patients who receive treatment after presenting to clinical services with symptoms or signs. Establishing whether this potential benefit is realized requires a balance sheet of the possible benefits and harms from screening (Chamberlain, 1984). Potential benefits include the improved outcome for cases detected through screening, as well as reassurance to individuals with true negative tests. Less radical treatment may sometimes be required following earlier diagnosis, benefitting patients and sometimes resulting in resource savings. The harms from screening may be experienced by true positive cases, including the longer period spent living with a diagnosis if prognosis is not altered, as well as overdiagnosis and overtreatment of borderline abnormalities. Harms also include false reassurance to those with false negative results, and the anxiety and morbidity from further testing of those with false positive results (Chamberlain, 1984).

Evaluating the outcomes of screening may be difficult because several biases may come into play when contrasting outcomes of screen-detected and clinically diagnosed cases, and these are particularly evident in cancer screening programmes (Box 14.3). In order to avoid biased estimates, the effectiveness of screening programmes should ideally be evaluated in randomized controlled trials that compare screened and unscreened populations. Where appropriate, mortality should

---

Box 14.3 Biases in evaluating screening outcomes

Lead-time bias: The lead time is the difference in time between detection by screening and the time at which a case might have been diagnosed clinically. Survival times for screen-detected cases will generally be longer by the length of the lead time.

Length bias: If a cancer population includes both rapidly progressing and slow-growing tumours, then slow-growing tumours will be over-represented among screen-detected cases because these tumours remain at a subclinical stage for longer.

Selection bias: Individuals who engage with screening programmes are usually in better health than those who decline screening invitations.

Overdiagnosis bias: Screening programmes may result in overdiagnosis of conditions that might not have presented clinically during an individual's lifetime.

---

be the preferred outcome measure rather than the duration of individual patient survival. Health economic evaluation should be conducted in parallel with the effectiveness study.

Screening trials may be difficult to conduct leading to problems of interpretation. Breast cancer screening has been the subject of several trials but there is still considerable debate concerning the possible benefits of screening (Gotzsche & Olsen, 2000). In the case of breast cancer, screening trials were generally conducted many years ago, before the recent improvements in breast cancer treatment. This makes it difficult to establish clear conclusions with respect to the benefits and harms of screening in the present day (Nelson et al., 2016). It is now recognized that while randomized trial evidence is important to inform decisions about the introduction of a screening programme, non-randomized interventional studies and observational study designs can be used to evaluate the impact and effectiveness of ongoing screening programmes (Lauby–Secretan et al., 2015).

Prostate cancer provides an instructive example (Box 14.4). In the European Randomized Study of Screening for Prostate Cancer (Schröder et al., 2009), use of prostate specific antigen (PSA) testing was associated with a 71% higher rate of prostate cancer diagnosis, with one additional cancer diagnosis for each 29 men screened. Mortality from prostate cancer was 19% lower in the screened trial arm, but 1,408 men would have to be screened and 49 men would have to be treated for prostate cancer to prevent one prostate cancer death. Policy recommendations in the UK and the USA are that PSA screening for prostate cancer should not be used because the limited benefits are likely to be outweighed by potential harms, including false positive results that require additional testing, overdiagnosis, overtreatment, and treatment complications.

Box 14.4 Prostate specific antigen screening and prostate cancer mortality in a randomized controlled trial: the European Randomized Study of Screening for Prostate Cancer

The European Randomized Study of Screening for Prostate Cancer (ERSPC) was set up in the early 1990s to determine whether a reduction in prostate cancer mortality could be achieved by prostate specific antigen (PSA) screening. The study recruited 182,000 men between the ages of 50 and 74 years, with a core age group of 55 to 69 years, through registries in seven European countries. The men were randomly assigned to a group that was offered PSA screening at an average of once every four years or to a control group. Men with positive PSA results were referred for a biopsy of the prostate. Treatment of prostate cancer was performed according to local policies and guidelines. The primary outcome was the rate of death from prostate cancer. Mortality follow-up was identical for the two study groups and ended on 31 December 2006.

Diagnosis of prostate cancer in men aged 55 to 69 years
Screening trial arm: 72,890 participants; 5,990 (8.2%) cancer diagnoses
Control trial arm: 89,353 participants; 4,307 (4.8%) cancer diagnoses

Screening resulted in 3.4% more men being diagnosed with prostate cancer. The number of men needed to be screened to yield one additional cancer diagnosis was 29.

Deaths from prostate cancer in men aged 55 to 69 years
Screening trial arm: 214 prostate cancer deaths (2.94 per 1,000 men screened)
Control trial arm: 326 prostate cancer deaths (3.65 per 1,000 men screened)

Screening resulted in 0.71 fewer prostate cancer deaths per 1,000 men screened. The number of men needed to screen to prevent one prostate cancer death was 1,408. Therefore, based on the results of this trial, 49 men (1,408/29) would require treatment for screen-detected prostate cancer to prevent one prostate cancer death.

US Preventive Task Force Recommendation (2018b)
'For men aged 55 to 69 years ... screening offers a small potential benefit of reducing the chance of death from prostate cancer in some men. However, many men will experience potential harms of screening, including false-positive results that require additional testing and possible prostate biopsy; overdiagnosis and overtreatment; and treatment complications, such as incontinence and erectile dysfunction.'

Source: data from Schröder, F.H., et al. (2009). 'Screening and prostate-cancer mortality in a random- ized European study'. *New England Journal of Medicine*, Vol. 360, pp. 1320–1328. Massachusetts Medical Society.

14.7 Screening programme management

A good screening programme has clear aims and objectives, is widely accepted and understood, is part of a clear pathway which works seamlessly with good communication to the screened population, has timely data transfer, and employs effective evaluation, surveillance, and monitoring. Screening pregnant women for human immunodeficiency virus (HIV) to prevent vertical transmission from mother to baby is an example of a successful programme in high-income countries. In the UK, this is conducted as part of a screening programme for infections that also includes hepatitis B and syphilis. A well- specified programme with timely follow-up and treatment with antiretroviral drugs can reduce vertical transmission and prevent cases of HIV in infants. In less well-resourced countries, HIV screening is also beginning to have an effect. UNICEF (2018) reported that in 2017 there were about 180,000 new HIV infections among children aged 0–14 years compared to 270,000 in 2010.

14.7.1 Monitoring and evaluation of programmes

Monitoring the performance of screening programmes is an essential element of ensuring that they deliver their potential and that expected benefits are achieved in practice. It is important to distinguish quality assurance, which should be part of all formal screening programmes, from external evaluation of outcomes. Quality assurance is a process of continual review of a programme against agreed expected outcomes. In England, quality assurance follows a process of defining the objectives for good a programme in terms of structure, process, and outcomes; translating these objectives into quality criteria; setting standards to be achieved for each criterion; as well as collating and publishing information on performance. Failures in screening programmes represent significant incidents. These must be investigated so as to identify and remedy the causes and communicate with affected individuals. It is essential that lessons are learned and changes made to existing programmes to prevent recurrence. In the context of managing an incident, this most important outcome can be neglected once media interest dies down and incident reports are completed.

More formal external evaluation usually focuses on the overall aims of a programme, including the extent to which it is achieving specific outcomes, such as impacts on mortality and life expectancy, or other outcomes. This may be done at a national or regional level in order to be able to demonstrate relevant impacts through comparisons with other areas. Different programmes have different challenges and cancer programmes, such as the one for breast cancer, highlight particular challenges.

Once implemented, screening programmes should be kept under review to determine whether they continue to be appropriate in a given context. Changes in disease epidemiology, the prevalence of risk factors, or developments in the possibility of primary prevention change the case for screening. Screening policy is evidence-informed, but political considerations also come into play; the discontinuation of screening programmes may be controversial and difficult to achieve if there is resistance from stakeholders and interest groups. The examples in Sections 14.7.2–14.7.4 are instructive.

14.7.2 Rubella screening

Rubella infection is widespread in many parts of the world and causes congenital anomalies when the mother is infected with rubella virus at a critical early stage of pregnancy. This may result in a range of defects including blindness. Rubella screening is performed in pregnancy in many countries, with vaccination offered after delivery to protect future pregnancies, while no protection is possible for the current pregnancy. In the UK, rubella testing in pregnancy has now been discontinued after review showed that it no longer met the criteria for a screening programme. Rubella infection in the UK is now infrequent and the condition has been classified as eliminated by the World Health Organization (WHO); rubella infection in pregnancy is very rare. Women who are fully immunized with the measles, mumps, and rubella (MMR) vaccine before becoming pregnant are protected against rubella in pregnancy. This provides an example of where the introduction of a primary prevention strategy, that achieved high levels of vaccination in childhood, has changed the epidemiology of the disease and made it possible to stop the screening programme.

14.7.3 Cervical cancer screening

Traditional cervical cancer screening programmes have employed cervical cytology testing. There is now increasing focus on human papilloma virus (HPV) infection as an antecedent of cervical cancer. In Scotland, HPV vaccination was introduced for girls in 2008. This has been followed by an 89% decline in cervical cytological abnormalities at age 20 years (Palmer et al., 2019). Recent evidence also shows that testing for HPV infection is a better way of identifying women at risk of cervical cancer than the cytology (smear) test. This new method of testing is in the process of being introduced in the UK as it has higher sensitivity for high-grade cervical intraepithelial neoplasia (CIN) than cytology and it also has a lower false negative rate than cytology (Castanon et al., 2018). In December 2017, Australia's National Cervical Screening Program (NCSP) underwent a renewal in which the two-yearly Pap smear programme for 18–69 year olds was replaced with five-yearly primary HPV testing (with partial HPV genotyping and liquid-based cytology triage) for 25–74-year-old women (Hall et al., 2019). This transition was informed by a modelled evaluation of the benefits, harms, and cost effectiveness of adopting the new screening programme (Cancer Council Australia, 2018).

14.7.4 Abdominal aortic aneurysm screening

Screening for abdominal aortic aneurysm (AAA) in men has been introduced in the UK and in Sweden, but there is an ongoing debate concerning its value. Initial cost-effectiveness analyses suggested that the cost per quality adjusted life year (QALY) gained was £43,485, with less than 30% probability of screening being cost-effective at a threshold of £30,000 per QALY (Ehlers et al., 2009). In recent years, the decline in prevalence of cardiovascular disease in general, and AAA in particular, may be making screening for this condition even less cost-effective (Johansson et al., 2018). A comparison of AAA mortality in areas in Sweden, with and without AAA screening, found that mortality decreased at similar rates in all areas irrespective of the programme. The adverse effects of screening, including false positive results, overdiagnosis, and avoidable surgery, make the balance in favour of screening debatable (Johansson et al., 2018).

14.8 Conclusions

The concept of screening is intuitively simple and appeals to the public, politicians, and professionals. The translation of this concept into a practical reality which can favourably impact on public health is a significant challenge, and one which requires good evidence, clear objectives, and ongoing monitoring and surveillance. Public engagement and acceptance are essential for a successful screening programme. Reports of successful ongoing programmes frequently receive less profile than proposed new programmes or problems with existing programmes where focus, attention, and evaluation have dropped away. This chapter has outlined key concepts, challenges, and examples to help with understanding this topic and providing an informed view on the subject.

References

Andermann, A., Blancquaert, I., Beauchamp, S., & Déry, V. (2008). Revisiting Wilson and Jungner in the genomic age: a review of screening criteria over the past 40 years. *Bull World Health Org*, 86, 317–319.

Australian Institute of Health and Welfare. (2017). *BreastScreen Australia Monitoring Report 2014–2015*. Cancer series no. 106. Cat. no. CAN 105. Canberra: Australian Institute of Health and Welfare.

Cancer Council Australia. (2018). *Modelled evaluation of the predicted benefits, harms and cost-effectiveness of the renewed National Cervical Screening Program (NCSP) in conjunction with these guideline recommendations.* Sydney, Australia: Cancer Council Australia.

Castanon, A., Landy, R., Pesola, F., Windridge, P., & Sasieni, P. (2018). Prediction of cervical cancer incidence in England, UK, up to 2040, under four scenarios: a modelling study. *Lancet Public Health*, 3, e34–e43.

Chamberlain, J.M. (1984). Which prescriptive screening programmes are worthwhile? *J Epidemiol Community Health*, 38, 270–277.

Ehlers, L., Overvad, K., Sørensen, J., Christensen, S., Bech, M., & Kjølby, M. (2009). Analysis of cost effectiveness of screening Danish men aged 65 for abdominal aortic aneurysm. *BMJ*, 338, b2243.

Gotzsche, P.C. & Olsen, O. (2000). Is screening for breast cancer with mammography justifiable? [see comments]. *Lancet*, 355, 129–134.

Hall, M.T., et al. (2019). The projected timeframe until cervical cancer elimination in Australia: a modelling study. *Lancet Public Health*, 4, e19–27.

Johansson, M., Zahl, P.H., Siersma, V., Jorgensen, K.J., Marklund, B., & Brodersen, J. (2018). Benefits and harms of screening men for abdominal aortic aneurysm in Sweden: a registry-based cohort study. *Lancet*, 391, 2441–2447.

Lauby–Secretan, B., et al. (2015). Breast-cancer screening—viewpoint of the IARC Working Group. *New Engl J Med*, 372, 2353–2358.

Raffle, A.E. & Gray, M. (2007). *Screening: Evidence and Practice*. Oxford: Oxford University Press.

Marteau, T.M., Dormandy, E., & Michie, S. (2001). A measure of informed choice. *Health Expect*, 4, 99–108.

McKeown, T. (1976). An approach to screening policies. *J R Coll Physicians Lond*, 10, 145–152.

Nelson, H.D., Fu, R., Cantor, A., Pappas, M., Daeges, M., & Humphrey, L. (2016). Effectiveness of breast cancer screening: systematic review and meta-analysis to update the 2009 U.S. Preventive Services Task Force recommendation effectiveness of breast cancer screening. *Ann Intern Med*, 164, 244–255.

Nuffield Council on Bioethics. (2018). *Whole Genome Sequencing of Babies*. London: Nuffield Council on Bioethics. Available at: https://www.nuffieldbioethics.org/publications/whole-genome-sequencing-of-babies [accessed 28 July 2019].

Orchard, J., Freedman, B., Lowres, N., & Neubeck, L. (2018). Atrial fibrillation: is there enough evidence to recommend opportunistic or systematic screening? *Int J Epidemiol*, 47, 1372–1378.

Pace, L.E. & Keating, N.L. (2014). A systematic assessment of benefits and risks to guide breast cancer screening decisions. *JAMA*, 311, 1327–1335.

Palmer, T., et al. (2019). Prevalence of cervical disease at age 20 after immunisation with bivalent HPV vaccine at age 12–13 in Scotland: retrospective population study. *BMJ*, 365, l1161.

Public Health England. (2019). *NHS Screening Timeline*. London: Public Health England.

Samavat, A. & Modell, B. (2004). Iranian national thalassaemia screening programme. *BMJ*, 329, 1134–1137.

Schröder, F.H., et al. (2009). Screening and prostate-cancer mortality in a randomized European study. *New Engl J Med*, 360, 1320–1328.

Streetly, A., Sisodia, R., Dick, M., Latinovic, R., Hounsell, K., & Dormandy, E. (2018). Evaluation of newborn sickle cell screening programme in England: 2010–2016. *Arch Dis Child*, 103, 648.

UK National Screening Committee. (2015). *Criteria for appraising the viability, effectiveness and appropriateness of a screening programme*. London: Department of Health and Social Care. Available at: https://www.gov.uk/government/publications/evidence-review-criteria-national-screening-programmes/criteria-for-appraising-the-viability-effectiveness-and-appropriateness-of-a-screening-programme [accessed 18 July 2019].

UK National Screening Committee. (2017). *Guidance: UK National Screening Committee evidence review process*. London: Department of Health and Social Care. Available at: https://www.gov.uk/government/publications/uk-nsc-evidence-review-process/uk-nsc-evidence-review-process [accessed 18 July 2019].

UNICEF. (2018). *Elimination of mother to child transmission. Progress made in reducing new HIV infections among children isn't fast enough.* Available at: https://data.unicef.org/topic/hivaids/emtct/ [accessed 18 July 2019].

US Commission on Chronic Illness. (1957). *Chronic Illness in the United States: Volume I. Prevention of Chronic Illness.* Cambridge, Mass.: Harvard University Press.

US Preventive Services Task Force. (2018a). Screening for atrial fibrillation With electrocardiography: US Preventive Services Task Force recommendation statement. *JAMA*, 320, 478–484.

US Preventive Services Task Force. (2018b). Screening for prostate cancer: US Preventive Services Task Force recommendation. *JAMA*, 319, 1901–1913.

Wald, D.S., Bestwick, J.P., Morris, J.K., Whyte, K., Jenkins, L., & Wald, N.J. (2016). Child–parent familial hypercholesterolemia screening in primary care. *New Engl J Med*, 375, 1628–1637.

15
Digital healthcare public health

Martin Gulliford, Edmund Jessop, and Lucy Yardley

15.1 Introduction

Over recent decades, the increasing accessibility, speed, and connectivity of computers has greatly increased the potential of population health and healthcare information. Data relevant to public health can be collected more efficiently; linked datasets provide 'big data' that can be readily analysed to yield new insights into public health and health system problems. The availability of computers has brought about a revolution in statistical methods, with the development of a new terminology including 'data science', 'predictive analytics', 'machine learning', and 'precision population health'. Population coverage and public engagement in the use of smartphones and other smart devices have increased rapidly. About 3.3 billion people worldwide had mobile access to the internet in 2018 (GSMA, 2018). In the UK, 66% of adults had a smartphone in 2015, including 90% of 16 to 24 year olds and 50% of 55 to 64 year olds; 90% of the population have access to the internet in their homes, with an average of two hours per day spent on the internet, most often using mobile phones (Ofcom, 2015). Smart devices provide portable computer operating systems to run software applications and connect to the internet, with potential for health-related intervention. The development of social media channels has contributed to the democratization of communication, with implications for public health.

This chapter reviews these developments. We focus on the future potential of digital technologies for population healthcare, but we also draw attention to problems that may arise from the uncritical application of technological innovations. We also draw attention to some ethical questions that may arise in digital public health.

15.2 Public health information and 'big data'

Public health intelligence has traditionally relied on analysis of vital registration data, including records of births and causes of death, as well as notifications and laboratory reports of infectious diseases, with the decennial census providing a population denominator. The replacement of paper-based records with computerized databases has increased the timeliness and accessibility of these data. Over time, public health information has been enriched through data collected by healthcare services. 'Routinely

Martin Gulliford, Edmund Jessop, and Lucy Yardley, *Digital healthcare public health* In: *Healthcare Public Health*. Edited by: Martin Gulliford and Edmund Jessop, Oxford University Press (2020). © Oxford University Press.
DOI: 10.1093/oso/9780198837206.003.0015.

collected data' include data collected primarily for administrative purposes, as well as electronic health records (EHRs) data that have been collected as part of the recording of clinical care. In the UK, almost the entire population is registered with a general practice, and most general practices employ computerized practice systems that maintain longitudinally continuous electronic records to document patients' healthcare, often over decades.

Primary care EHRs have now been collected into databases of longitudinal anonymized records such as the Clinical Practice Research Datalink (CPRD). The CPRD includes data for some 7% of general practices in the UK from 1990 to the present, with an average registered population of about 4.5 million and nearly 90 million person years of follow-up (Herrett et al., 2015). Primary care EHR data have been analysed to make many important contributions to clinical epidemiology and public health as, for example, in the monitoring of childhood obesity trends, analysing drug safety, or the impact of population health campaigns. EHRs are now also being utilized in interventional research (van Staa et al., 2014) and in health economic evaluations (Hazra et al., 2019).

In recent years, EHR data resources have been strengthened by linking multiple data sources. CPRD data are now linked to mortality data, deprivation statistics, hospital episode statistics, and disease registry records for cancer and myocardial infarction. Data linkage has advantages in terms of improving case ascertainment and providing additional detail concerning diagnosis, management, and resource use. Box 15.1 presents an example in which linked data were used to improve the

---

Box 15.1 Data linkage and myocardial infarction ascertainment

A study of myocardial infarction (Herrett et al., 2013) found that by linking data from various data sources, it was possible to obtain improved estimates of the incidence and case fatality of myocardial infarction. The study included 21,482 patients with acute myocardial infarction in England between 2003 and 2009. They were identified in four linked electronic health record sources: primary care, hospital admissions, the disease registry (Myocardial Ischaemia National Audit Project), and the national mortality register (cause-specific mortality data).

Only 5,561 (31.0%) patients were recorded in all three sources, and 11,482 (63.9%) in at least two sources. The crude incidence of acute myocardial infarction was underestimated by 25–50% using one source compared with using all three sources. Compared with acute myocardial infarction defined in the disease registry, the positive predictive value of acute myocardial infarction recorded in primary care was 92.2% (95% confidence interval 91.6–92.8%) and in hospital admissions was 91.5% (95% confidence interval 90.8–92.1%).

The study concluded that each data source missed a substantial proportion (25–50%) of myocardial infarction events. Using linked data sources is important to avoid biased estimates of the incidence and outcome of myocardial infarction.

ascertainment of myocardial infarction for population-based studies. Missing data are an important issue in the analysis of EHRs because these data are a by-product of clinical healthcare delivery and are usually analysed for a purpose for which they were not collected. Missing values in health records data are typically 'missing not at random'; data values are only recorded if clinicians see a reason to document them (Agniel et al., 2018). The simple act of recording a laboratory test result may be associated with the patient's health outcome regardless of the test value (Agniel et al., 2018). It is important to be aware that this type of bias may be propagated through any 'big data' analysis (Prosperi et al., 2018).

Evolution in the use of data has also been occurring in the study of the determinants of health. Early area-based measures of deprivation in England included the Townsend score, which focused on the population census as a single data source, and employed only four metrics: non-car ownership, non-home ownership, household overcrowding, and unemployment (Townsend et al., 1985). By contrast, the 2015 Indices of Multiple Deprivation score combined information across seven domains of deprivation: income, employment, education, health, crime, housing, and the environment (Ministry of Housing, Communities, and Local Government, 2015). Each domain drew on analysis of data from multiple sources to generate a basket of domain indicators, with the 'health' domain including indicators for years of potential life lost, disability, acute morbidity, and mood and anxiety disorders. The financial services company Experian (2019) developed a consumer segmentation tool known as 'Mosaic', drawing on a wide range of data sources including more than 450 different variables. The Mosaic tool divides the UK population into 15 sociodemographic groups and 66 discrete types. This segmentation tool is primarily designed to inform commercial marketing strategies, but applications in public health have also been explored. For example, an exploratory study found that the healthcare costs of multimorbidity patients varied across Mosaic groups (Doos et al., 2013).

We are now entering a new phase of 'big data' collection and analysis. Most individuals now generate an electronic trace of their activities through use of customer loyalty cards and financial services cards that track their purchases; smart meters that monitor their use of utility services; smartphones and monitoring devices that reveal their location, as well as engagement in leisure-time physical activity; and use of social media channels that enables mapping of their social networks. These new types of data have the potential to be analysed for public health benefit. For example, smart-meter data could be used to analyse fuel poverty; and data about people's movements could be used to provide improved estimates of exposure to atmospheric pollution. However, the same data could be employed for private gain, with negative implications for public health, if they are used to enhance the marketing of harmful products including tobacco, alcohol, and high-sugar, high-fat foods. 'Big data' analysis has the potential to compromise core ethical principles including autonomy, confidentiality, fairness, and non-maleficence; appropriate governance and safeguards are essential.

15.3 Data science and population healthcare

Developments in computation have driven a revolution in statistical data analysis techniques (Efron & Hastie, 2016). The availability of computers has made it possible to implement a wide range of sophisticated approaches to data analysis, informed by both frequentist and Bayesian thinking. Whereas the frequentist approach estimates the probability of obtaining study data under the null hypothesis, the Bayesian approach allows us to estimate the probability of the study hypothesis given the data that has been observed in a study. The frequentist P-value is prone to misinterpretation, especially when an arbitrary cut-point such as P<0.05 is used (Greenland et al., 2016), and this approach to interpretation should no longer be used (Amrhein et al., 2019).

Computer-age statistical techniques are increasingly informing data analyses conducted in academic, public sector, and commercial settings. Data science methods have transformed the activity of routine data analysis into a cutting-edge area of scientific enquiry. This has been accompanied by a growing debate concerning the relative roles of humans and computers in designing and controlling data analyses (Beam & Kohane, 2018).

15.3.1 Machine learning and artificial intelligence

One area of healthcare in which computers might perform better than humans is in interpreting imaging data. Box 15.2 provides one example in which machine learning was used to read digital retinal photographs for signs of diabetic retinopathy. This raises the possibility that screening programmes might use computer-aided techniques to read screening tests in order to maintain quality and optimize

---

Box 15.2 Machine learning and diabetic retinopathy detection

Gulshan et al. (2016) analysed digital retinal images of 4,997 diabetic patients. In order to provide reference data for analysis, the images were graded by ophthalmologists for the presence of diabetic retinopathy. The images and report data were used to develop a machine-learning algorithm that classified the severity of diabetic retinopathy based on the pixel data contained in the fundus images. The algorithm represented a large network-like mathematical function with many parameters known as a neural network. The algorithm was found to have 97% sensitivity and 93% specificity for classifying diabetic retinopathy, with a negative predictive value of about 99.8%, indicating that in 1,000 negative screens there might be two false negative results. The study authors suggested that this algorithm could now be evaluated in clinical practice with a view to using it to improve patients' care and treatment outcomes compared with conventional management.

test performance. Similar techniques are now being developed across many areas of healthcare. Initial promising results suggest that machine-learning techniques might be used in future to automate important tasks in healthcare, potentially replacing human analytical capacities, with possible efficiency gains.

There are significant challenges to be addressed before this potential can be realized. Machine-learning approaches require large amounts of data, often with millions of records, before a model can be developed to address a complex problem, and suitable amounts of data of sufficient quality may not always be available (Wang et al., 2019). Machine-learning models may not be transferable between different data-collection systems: that is, they may lack interoperability. Models may not be easy to interpret: humans will normally provide reasons for arriving at a particular conclusion, but this may not be the case for machine-learning algorithms, which might offer only the estimated probability of a conclusion without supporting justification (Wang et al., 2019).

Machine-learning approaches have received criticism from several quarters. A systematic review of studies that compared prediction modelling using a range of machine-learning methods with traditional logistic regression modelling techniques did not find evidence that machine-learning methods resulted in prediction models with better performance. However, the conclusions of the review cannot be considered definitive because the poor methodological quality and incomplete reporting of the studies suggested that better-conducted studies might yield different results. From the artificial intelligence perspective, the kinds of problems that can be solved through machine learning are considered to have a low level of complexity because they concern statistical association rather than causal reasoning Pearl (2018).

In a recent commentary, Beam and Kohane (2018) suggested that human-led and machine-led data analysis and decision making should be viewed as a spectrum. Human-led analysis works well for small datasets including tens of observations. When there are hundreds or thousands of observations, computer-aided regression modelling techniques will generally be required, but the outputs from these techniques are familiar, transparent, and straightforward to interpret. As the size of a dataset increases, the contribution of human decision making is reduced and machine-led decision making becomes more important, requiring use of techniques like random forests and neural networks when datasets have millions or billions of observations. These techniques produce algorithms that may be difficult to understand but will function as 'black boxes' (Beam & Kohane, 2018) to be applied to healthcare and public health. At the stage of application into practice, it will be important to evaluate whether an algorithm is providing valid results that are consistent with public health objectives and with social and ethical values.

15.3.2 Geographical information systems

Advances in computation have made it possible to analyse spatial data extremely efficiently. Geographical information systems (GISs) now have several applications in healthcare planning and operational delivery, as well as in public health more broadly. In general, the further away patients are from a healthcare facility, the less they will use it. This creates an obligation for healthcare planners to monitor usage. The theoretical ideal is that two patients with identical clinical conditions should have the same probability of treatment regardless of location. That ideal cannot be measured, and the commonest proxy is to examine access rates per million resident population in a geographic area. One key decision is the size of geographical unit chosen for analysis: too large, and important variation is obscured; too small, and the number of events in each unit becomes sparse (Coles et al., 2012).

GISs can be used to plan the location of healthcare facilities, typically to minimize travel for patients in time-critical services such as trauma, vascular surgery, and cadaveric organ transplant. This may lead to suggestions for placing new facilities to improve access (Webb et al., 2019) or for reducing the number of facilities in an overprovided jurisdiction, while still ensuring timely access. Less dramatically, identifying zones where hospital catchments overlap in densely populated areas may prompt discussions about preferred providers: multiplicity and choice is good but not conducive to clear, efficient pathways between primary and secondary care. GISs have also been used operationally, to deploy limited ambulance resources dynamically across wide areas: ambulances start the day spread evenly across the region but, as each ambulance is called to a task, all other ambulances shift their locations to fill the gaps.

15.3.3 'Precision public health'

A third area where new analytical techniques might be applied is in risk prediction and population segmentation. Risk prediction and risk stratification are established techniques in clinical medicine. The Framingham Risk Score represented an early attempt to develop an algorithm to identify individuals at elevated risk of cardiovascular diseases who might benefit from risk-reduction interventions (Anderson et al., 1991). The electronic Frailty Index (eFI) represents a method for classifying older people into differing levels of frailty based on information about symptoms, signs, disabilities, diseases, and laboratory measurements recorded in their EHRs (Clegg et al., 2016). Greater frailty is associated with increased risk of hospital admissions, fractures, and mortality. Machine-learning techniques are now being applied to 'big data' with the aim of developing more sophisticated risk-stratification tools through linking EHRs with genomic and other laboratory data.

Existing disease classifications are based on phenotypic features such as the type of organ affected or the pathological appearances. Linking laboratory data with phenotypic data from health records has the potential to reveal more fundamental disease classifications based on molecular mechanisms. Individuals and groups may sometimes have a molecular make-up that favours a response to a specific intervention. These ideas have contributed to the evolution of 'stratified medicine' or 'precision medicine', and have their counterpart in the concept of 'precision public health', which incorporates the notion of delivering the 'right intervention to the right population at the right time' (Khoury, 2018).

Machine learning applied to 'big data' has the potential to estimate risks more precisely, identifying targets for public health interventions. Examples include use of classification trees to identify population subgroups who are at high risk of having undiagnosed hypertension (Collins & Winkleby, 2002) or not having completed mammographic screening (Gomez et al., 2007) that might benefit from targeted intervention. Population segmentation is also being used by healthcare providers to improve management of both resources and patients. Population segmentation algorithms have been developed to aid the identification of 'high-need, high-cost' patients who might benefit from distinct care strategies (Yan et al., 2019).

Many authors have drawn attention to potential problems in the 'precision public health' approach. Risk prediction may present ethical problems if used to present the individualized risks of having a stigmatized condition, such as substance abuse or a sexually transmitted infection, or used to define eligibility or potentially enable discrimination in access to healthcare in an insurance-based system. Notions of 'precision' should not distract attention from the important stratifier of social inequality, which there may be a lack of political will to address (Chowkwanyun et al., 2018). Universal intervention strategies are often more effective in public health because a majority of cases of disease may arise in the larger number who are intermediate or at low risk, rather than the smaller group at high risk (Chowkwanyun et al., 2018). Finally, a relevant insight from behaviour change research is that informing people of their level of risk seldom changes their behaviour, unless they believe the risk is imminent and very serious and they are confident they can make a low-cost response to avert it effectively. This observation draws attention to the importance of considering the interface between human behaviour and digital technologies as tools for public health intervention.

15.4 Digital interventions and population healthcare

Digital technology provides many opportunities for public health and healthcare intervention through measuring and changing the behaviour of healthcare providers and users. Digital interventions may be employed in a wide range of contexts including promoting practitioners' implementation of evidence-based interventions and recommended standards of clinical practice, increasing patients' adherence with healthcare interventions and encouraging self-care, as well as supporting changes in health-related behaviour across the population at risk. Box 15.3 provides an example of electronic intervention from antimicrobial resistance research.

As we noted earlier, individual-level behavioural data collected automatically by healthcare information systems and smart devices can be aggregated into 'big data'

> ## Box 15.3 Digital intervention in a data-enabled trial
>
> The REDUCE trial was a cluster randomized trial embedded in the UK Clinical Practice Research Datalink (CPRD). The trial aimed to reduce unnecessary use of antibiotics for respiratory infections in primary care (Gulliford et al., 2019). The electronically delivered interventions included a webinar, computer-delivered decision-support tools that were activated during consultations for respiratory illness, and monthly antibiotic prescribing reports prepared from analyses of electronic health records data.
>
> Development of the antimicrobial stewardship intervention drew on social cognitive theory, self-determination theory, and qualitative interviews with 31 prescribers to refine prototype versions of interventions. The primary outcome was the rate of antibiotic prescriptions for respiratory tract infections, which was obtained from analysis of primary care electronic health records. Episodes of serious bacterial complications were evaluated as safety outcomes.
>
> The trial included 41 antimicrobial stewardship practices (323,155 patient years) and 38 usual-care practices (259,520 patient years). The adjusted antibiotic prescribing rate ratio was 0.88 (0.78–0.99, P=0.04), respectively, with prescribing rates of 98.7 per 1,000 patient years for antimicrobial stewardship (31,907 prescriptions) and 107.6 per 1,000 patient years for usual care (27,923 prescriptions). There was also no evidence of an increase in serious bacterial complications (0.92, 0.74–1.13).
>
> The study concluded that electronically delivered interventions, integrated into practice workflow, result in moderate reductions of antibiotic prescribing for respiratory tract infections in adults, which are likely to be of importance for public health.

sets, representing data from large numbers of digital technology users. This makes it possible to map a range of individual behaviour patterns and their changes over time, and to identify personal and contextual factors that modify these behaviours. Machine-learning techniques can be exploited to help analyse this information and develop digital interventions and information resources that may be presented to healthcare providers and service users; effects on health-related behaviour can be analysed in pragmatic trials and real-world experiments (Hekler et al., 2016). These new methods of digital assessment, analysis, and intervention may in turn inform new ways of understanding and theorizing health- and healthcare-related behaviour.

Increasingly, digital interventions are being developed to provide behaviour-change prompts precisely when and where they are needed. Health professionals may be provided with computer-delivered prompts that present information to support clinical decision making for the particular context of their consultation. Patients with long-term conditions may be prompted to engage in activity at home after a digital device has detected a period of extended inactivity. These 'just-in-time' adaptive interventions (JITAIs) have the potential to take into account user characteristics, their environments, and individual needs on a dynamic basis (Spruijt–Metz et al., 2015).

Intervention through digital technology may also be valuable for global health because of the rapidly expanding coverage and low marginal cost of allowing additional users to access existing digital interventions. Digital technologies make it possible to share population health intervention strategies with low- and middle-income countries at low cost (Muñoz, 2010). The rapid uptake of mobile phone technology worldwide, even among people with limited incomes and literacy, is reducing existing barriers to global use of digital tools and interventions. Future research needs to evaluate the extent to which digital interventions may need to be adapted for people from different socioeconomic and ethnic backgrounds (Latulippe et al., 2017).

A common problem with many digital interventions to date is that there is often low usage and rapid drop-out—because these interventions are typically accessed independently by users, without the support and encouragement of healthcare workers. There is consensus that to improve engagement with digital interventions it is necessary to employ user-centred approaches to intervention development (Yardley et al., 2016). These approaches include user-centred design and participatory co-design. Stakeholders and target users are involved throughout the design process, with the aim of maximizing the accessibility, usability, and appropriateness of an intervention in order to improve reach and engagement. User-centred approaches are widely used in the field of human–computer interaction; sometimes the focus is simply on testing the usability of basic functions (e.g. ease of navigation) and the user interface, but often the scope includes a broader consideration of user needs, preferences, and lifestyle. The Person-Based Approach is a user-centred approach that originated in the discipline of health psychology and seeks to ensure that interventions are not just attractive and easy to use but are experienced as personally relevant and convincing, and provide support for offline behaviour change (for example, by increasing motivation and confidence) (Yardley et al., 2015). The Person-Based Approach draws on qualitative research methods to understand users' beliefs, capabilities, and context, which inform the co-design of the intervention. Further qualitative research, combined with stakeholder co-design, is then used to refine the intervention in order to maximize acceptability and feasibility—and hence uptake, engagement, and effectiveness.

A common method of improving the personal relevance and therefore usage of interventions is to 'tailor' the content to the user. Tailoring involves collecting information about the user (for example, their characteristics, concerns, current behaviour, or preferences) and using this information to deliver personalized advice. For example, a digital smoking-cessation intervention tailored messages to users based on their reported smoking history and patterns, home environment, and levels of stress and coping. These high levels of personalization led to better perceived personal relevance of messages, more engagement, and higher rates of smoking cessation (Strecher et al., 2008). However, tailoring digital interventions increases their complexity and cost, but does not always increase effectiveness. More research is needed to understand when and why tailoring is needed and useful. Further research is also required to understand how much engagement is actually necessary to achieve positive outcomes, since some very brief but well-targeted interventions may be effective. The type and amount of intervention usage needed to achieve positive outcomes—which has been termed 'effective engagement'—is likely to differ between interventions, and can only be established by examining both online usage patterns and actual behaviour change (Yardley et al., 2016).

Traditional behavioural models, methods, and theories have been applied success-fully to developing digital interventions, and new models and approaches are rapidly being developed to suit the specific opportunities and challenges of digital technology. However, there remain many important unanswered questions (Fairburn & Patel, 2017). The new theoretical frameworks and methods that have been proposed have not yet been empirically tested or validated. There is great excitement about the po-tential of digital technology to trigger support for healthy behaviour when and where it is needed, but there is not yet strong evidence that this will have important positive effects on health. Many thousands of health-related web- and phone-based applica-tions ('apps') have been developed to support individual behaviour change, but most of these lack any evidence of effectiveness. Moreover, apps that rely on supporting individual self-regulation of behaviour risk increasing health inequalities, since those with less education and income are known to be less likely to engage with and benefit from them, despite their greater health needs.

To achieve better population health we may need to turn our attention to creating a digital environment that supports health automatically, by prompting and nudging attitudes and behaviour in a more healthy direction—in the same way that advertisers are successfully using the digital environment to prompt consumer choices. To do so, it will be necessary to work closely with large-scale public- and private-sector pro-viders of digital services, as they have the requisite infrastructure and can reach large sectors of the population.

15.5 Digital communication and population healthcare

In the health field, the rapid and open transfer of information through the internet has altered the balance of power between consumers and professionals whose role, influence, and prestige has traditionally been supported by their controlled access to specialist knowledge (Smith & Graham, 2017). This shift has had benefits in terms of supporting patients' autonomy in making decisions that affect their health, enabling more informed choices in healthcare. However, the internet also offers immediate ac-cess to information that may not be quality-assured, sometimes lacking a basis in evi-dence or being compromised by conflicts of interest.

The role of social media in the propagation of anti-vaccine messaging is instructive. Initial reports that cast doubt on the safety of the measles, mumps, and rubella (MMR) vaccine were circulated through traditional scientific and print media, but in recent years, social media have provided an important channel for the dissemination of anti-vaccine messages (Box 15.4). Smith and Graham (2017) analysed the role of

---

Box 15.4 Social media and the spread of vaccine information

In March 2016, an illegal vaccine distribution network was discovered in China's Shandong province, where approximately two million doses of unrefrigerated (often expired) vaccine had been dispensed over a period of five years, causing public concern. Gu et al. (2017) investigated the reporting of the incident by administering a questionnaire to 26,000 people. Their study showed that 78% of respondents received information about the vaccine incident exclusively from social media, with most people gaining access to information spread rapidly through informal social media communications before official, substantiated reports were released. The authors concluded that public health professionals and policy makers should develop the capacity to act openly and promptly through social media to address public concerns and provide transparent and up-to-date information.

Facebook in the anti-vaccination movement and showed how social media sites play a supporting role in propagating and sustaining informal movements that promote strongly held but not well-evidenced views against vaccination. These are often linked to wider distrust of authority and existing social structures. Consequently, people searching for information about vaccination on the internet may encounter false as well as true information that may shape their views and influence their decision on whether or not to vaccinate. Social media communication may also contribute to political campaigns against vaccination (Smith & Graham, 2017). In social media communication concerning water fluoridation, anti-fluoridation views outnumber pro-fluoridation views by between five and sixty-fold (Mertz & Allukian, 2014), leading to underappreciation of the possible benefits that water fluoridation offers and its potentially large impact on inequalities in dental health.

Miscommunication in relation to public health messaging is part of a wider societal concern with politically motivated manipulation and false communication through social media. At the time of writing, social media platforms have become more aware of the reputational harm that springs from false messages and have engaged in self-regulation, with YouTube, Facebook, and Instagram committing to ban groups, pages, and advertisements that spread false information about vaccines. The Chief Executive of Facebook also made a more general call for greater governmental regulation of social media platforms. There is also a need for the public health and scientific communities to engage in direct communication with wide public audiences to ensure open, transparent, and timely communication of the benefits and risks associated with vaccination.

15.6 Concluding remarks

The rapid development and application of new information technologies in the 'Information Age' is having a major impact on all aspects of economic activity and societal functioning. Public health needs to embrace these changes and be at the forefront of efforts to harness these new technologies to improve population health and reduce inequalities. Some of the traditional methods of public health, including older statistical analysis methods, will be replaced by new and more powerful techniques. Other methods, such as disease mapping, will be developed to higher levels of sophistication through more advanced analytical techniques applied to larger and more complex datasets. The reach of digital technology should make it available to a wide global population, but there remain significant barriers to uptake, engagement, and universal dissemination. Nonetheless, there is great optimism that digital technology will soon transform our ability to support providers and patients in their management of health and health problems. Realizing this potential will require new approaches that involve behavioural scientists, clinicians, data scientists, service users, and specialists in informatics and software engineering (Schueller et al., 2013). We have already learned that it is essential to work closely with intended users and stakeholders to ensure that digital resources are accessible, usable, and useful. In order to implement interventions widely and reap the benefits of carrying out large-scale real-world research, we also need to work with commercial partners, healthcare providers, and experts in business, economics, and policy. This will require collaboration and communication with broad groups of experts, which is itself a new but essential venture.

References

Agniel, D., Kohane, I.S., & Weber, G.M. (2018). Biases in electronic health record data due to processes within the healthcare system: retrospective observational study. *BMJ*, 361, k 1479.

Amrhein, V., Greenland, S., & McShane, B. (2019). Scientists rise up against statistical significance. *Nature*, 567, 305–307.

Anderson, K.M., Odell, P.M., Wilson, P.W., & Kannel, W.B. (1991). Cardiovascular disease risk profiles. *Am Heart J*, 121, 293–298.

Beam, A.L. & Kohane, I.S. (2018). Big data and machine learning in health care. *JAMA*, 319, 1317–1318.

Chowkwanyun, M., Bayer, R., & Galea, S. (2018). 'Precision' public health—between novelty and hype. *New Engl J Med*, 379, 1398–1400.

Clegg, A., et al. (2016). Development and validation of an electronic frailty index using routine primary care electronic health record data. *Age Ageing*, 45, 353–360.

Coles, S., Haire, K., Kenny, T., & Jessop, E.G. (2012). Monitoring access to nationally commissioned services in England. *Orphanet J Rare Dis*, 7, 85.

Collins, R. & Winkleby, M.A. (2002). African American women and men at high and low risk for hypertension: a signal detection analysis of NHANES III, 1988–1994. *Prev Med*, 35, 303–312.

Doos, L., Uttley, J., Onyia, I., Iqbal, Z., Jones, P.W., & Kadam, U.T. (2013). Mosaic segmentation, COPD and CHF multimorbidity and hospital admission costs: a clinical linkage study. *J Public Health*, 36, 317–324.

Efron, B. & Hastie, T. (2016). *Computer Age Statistical Inference: Algorithms, Evidence, and Data Science*. New York: Cambridge University Press.

Experian. (2019). *Mosaic Digital. Comprehensive Insight into the Digital Behaviour of Your Consumers*. Nottingham: Experian.

Fairburn, C.G. & Patel, V. (2017). The impact of digital technology on psychological treatments and their dissemination. *Behav Res Ther*, 88, 19–25.

Gomez, S.L., Tan, S., Keegan, T.H., & Clarke, C.A. (2007). Disparities in mammographic screening for Asian women in California: a cross-sectional analysis to identify meaningful groups for targeted intervention. *BMC Cancer*, 7, 201.

Greenland, S., et al. (2016). Statistical tests, P values, confidence intervals, and power: a guide to misinterpretations. *Eur J Epidemiol*, 31, 337–350.

GSMA. (2018). *State of Mobile Internet Connectivity 2018*. London: GSMA.

Gu, Z., Su, J., Badger, P., Li, X., Zhang, L., & Zhang, E. (2017). A vaccine crisis in the era of social media. *Nat Sci Rev*, 5, 8–10.

Gulliford, M.C., et al. (2019). Effectiveness and safety of electronically delivered pre-scribing feedback and decision support on antibiotic use for respiratory illness in primary care: REDUCE cluster randomised trial. *BMJ*, 364, l236.

Gulshan, V., et al. (2016). Development and validation of a deep learning algorithm for detec-tion of diabetic retinopathy in retinal fundus photographs. *JAMA*, 316, 2402–2410.

Hazra, N.C., Rudisill, C., & Gulliford, M.C. (2019). Developing the role of electronic health records in economic evaluation. *Eur J Health Econ*, 20(8), 1117–1121. doi: 10.1007/s10198-019-01042-5.

Hekler, E.B., et al. (2016). Agile science: creating useful products for behavior change in the real world. *Transl Behav Med*, 6, 317–328.

Herrett, E., et al. (2013). Completeness and diagnostic validity of recording acute myocardial infarction events in primary care, hospital care, disease registry, and national mortality re-cords: cohort study. *BMJ*, 346, f2350

Herrett, E., et al. (2015). Data resource profile: Clinical Practice Research Datalink (CPRD). *Int J Epidemiol*, 44, 827–836.

Khoury, M.J. (2018). *Precision Public Health. What Is It?* Atlanta, Ga.: Centers for Disease Control. Available at: https://blogs.cdc.gov/genomics/2018/05/15/precision-public-health-2/ [accessed 16 July 2019].

Latulippe, K., Hamel, C., & Giroux, D. (2017). Social health inequalities and ehealth: a litera-ture review with qualitative synthesis of theoretical and empirical studies. *J Med Internet Res*, 19, e136.

Mertz, A. & Allukian, M. (2014). Community water fluoridation on the internet and social media. *J Mass Dent Soc*, 63, 32–36.

Ministry of Housing, Communities & Local Government. (2015). *English Indices of Deprivation 2015*. London: Ministry of Housing, Communities & Local Government. Available at: https://www.gov.uk/government/statistics/english-indices-of-deprivation-2015 [ac-cessed 16 July 2019].

Muñoz, R.F. (2010). Using evidence-based internet interventions to reduce health disparities worldwide. *J Med Internet Res*, 12, e60.

Ofcom. (2015). *The UK Is Now a Smartphone Society*. London: Ofcom.

Pearl, J, M.D. (2018). *The Book of Why*. London: Penguin Books.

Prosperi, M., Min, J.S., Bian, J., & Modave, F. (2018). Big data hurdles in precision medicine and precision public health. *BMC Med Inform Decis Mak*, 18, 139.

Schueller, S.M., Muñoz, R.F., & Mohr, D.C. (2013). Realizing the potential of behavioral inter-vention technologies. *Curr Dir Psychol Sci*, 22, 478–483.

Smith, N. & Graham, T. (2017). Mapping the anti-vaccination movement on Facebook. *Inf Commun Soc*, 22, 1310–27.

Spruijt–Metz, D., et al. (2015). Building new computational models to support health behavior change and maintenance: new opportunities in behavioral research. *Transl Behav Med*, 5, 335–346.

Strecher, V.J., et al. (2008). The role of engagement in a tailored web-based smoking cessation program: randomized controlled trial. *J Med Internet Res*, 10, e36.

Townsend, P., Simpson, D., & Tibbs, N. (1985). Inequalities in health in the city of Bristol: a preliminary review of statistical evidence. *Int J Health Serv*, 15, 637–663.

van Staa, T.-P., et al. (2014). The opportunities and challenges of pragmatic point-of-care randomised trials using routinely collected electronic records: evaluations of two exemplar trials. *Health Technol Assess*, 18, 1–146.

Wang, F., Casalino, L.P., & Khullar, D. (2019). Deep learning in medicine—promise, progress, and challenges. *JAMA Intern Med*, 179, 293–294.

Webb, G.J., et al. (2019). Proximity to transplant center and outcome among liver transplant patients. *Am J Transplant*, 19, 208–220.

Yan, J., et al. (2019). Applying machine learning algorithms to segment high-cost patient populations. *J Gen Intern Med*, 34, 211–217.

Yardley, L., Morrison, L., Bradbury, K., & Muller, I. (2015). The person-based approach to intervention development: application to digital health-related behavior change interventions. *J Med Internet Res*, 17, e30.

Yardley, L., et al. (2016). Understanding and promoting effective engagement with digital behavior change interventions. *Am J Prev Med*, 51, 833–842.

16
Healthcare public health in disasters and emergencies

Edmund Jessop

16.1 Introduction

This chapter outlines the public health role in preparing health systems for the occurrence of emergencies and disasters. Disasters and emergencies are inevitable but also unpredictable in terms of when and where they will occur, who will be affected, and the nature and duration of the impacts. Consequently, it is important for public health services and health systems to prepare a plan that can be adapted to the circumstances of each incident.

In this chapter, the terms 'disaster', 'emergency', and 'incident' will be used interchangeably. In a simple definition, an emergency is any incident which threatens to overwhelm local capacity. This is consistent with the United Nations Office for Disaster Risk Reduction (UNDRR) definition of a disaster as 'a serious disruption of the functioning of a community or a society at any scale due to hazardous events interacting with conditions of exposure, vulnerability and capacity, leading to one or more of the following: human, material, economic and environmental losses and impacts' (UNDRR, 2020). Emergencies and disasters may have many different causes. Natural disasters include acute events like earthquakes, floods, hurricanes, volcanic eruptions and avalanches, as well as more insidious events like droughts and famines. Infectious disease outbreaks and epidemics represent biological emergencies that may often emerge from natural disasters. Technological disasters may include transport accidents or industrial accidents, while societal emergencies include civil disturbances, terrorist attacks, wars, and nuclear accidents (Roberts and Brennan, 2015). However, the apparent distinction between 'natural' and 'man-made' disasters is sometimes artificial. Wildfires are a natural phenomenon that can be aggravated by human actions. Climate change has its origins in human actions but may be leading to more frequent and widespread natural disasters. The scale and severity of a disaster can be gauged in terms of the number of people likely to be affected, the extent of geographical spread, or the potential impact on a population. In the Salisbury nerve agent attack in 2018, only a few individuals were directly affected but a full emergency response was required because of the severity of the impact and the potential for more widespread harm.

Edmund Jessop, *Healthcare public health in disasters and emergencies* In: *Healthcare Public Health*. Edited by: Martin Gulliford and Edmund Jessop, Oxford University Press (2020). © Oxford University Press.
DOI: 10.1093/oso/9780198837206.003.0016.

Planning and responding to disasters and emergencies must take place at multiple levels. In the 2009 influenza epidemic, the World Health Organization produced guidelines at global level for influenza pandemic preparedness and response; national governments produced plans for their own countries, adapting international models to their own circumstances. Planning also took place at local level to ensure that local services adapted to the expected surge in demand.

Emergency plans must also encompass many sectors of society. In this chapter, our main focus is on health services and public health responses, but these must be coordinated with the actions of other emergency services, local and national governments, the private sector, as well as third-sector organizations and the public. Hospitals have a strong tradition of planning for disasters or 'mass casualty incidents' as they are often called. The focus on hospital and 'casualties' implies a large number of people with traumatic injury in need of immediate life-saving treatment. These efforts have proved invaluable in saving lives in incidents all over the globe, but they also highlight the need for plans to extend far wider than the context of a single hospital or a single injury-causing event.

As a minimum, any plan for a disaster or emergency needs to include the whole *healthcare* system—from first responders, through ambulance services, primary care, surgical and other hospital care, to long-term rehabilitation. However, the plan also needs to show how hospitals will interact with each other and with agencies such as police, fire, and civic authorities; with agencies which provide social care including shelter, food, and water; and, depending on the emergency, with a wide range of other organizations such as radiation protection or chemical hazard specialists.

Emergency preparedness can be viewed as a cyclical process with several distinct phases. One framework identifies the required actions as 'Plan, Prepare, Respond, Recover, Report' (Figure 16.1). Some frameworks also include disaster risk reduction, focusing on the prevention of disasters, and disaster mitigation, focusing on reducing the impact of disasters, which are mostly beyond the scope of this chapter.

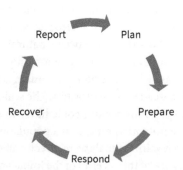

Figure 16.1 The plan–prepare–respond–recover–report framework for emergency preparedness.

16.2 Emergency planning

The planning phase includes risk assessment and consideration of all possible disasters that may occur within the jurisdiction of a health authority or organization. As we will see, this phase includes consideration of who leads the planning and how the plans of separate organizations interlock in order to complement rather than conflict with each other. The planning process is usually incremental, drawing on and refining previous plans that may already be in existence. A valid plan should consider all relevant potential disasters and emergencies, and all serious potential outcomes. After the long list is compiled, a framework of priorities for risk management is needed to guide decisions on what time and resources should be allocated to preparing for each specific risk, drawing on estimates of incident severity and likelihood of occurrence. In England, for example, earthquakes severe enough to cause damage are effectively unknown, so it would not be sensible to devote resources to earthquake planning; whereas in New Zealand and many other countries, earthquake planning is essential. In contrast, every health system now needs to prepare for the large numbers of traumatic injury that might be caused by a terrorist incident, even though these are infrequent, or for a major fire disaster that might overwhelm the burn-care facilities of an entire country.

The identification of potential disasters may point to possibilities for prevention, though responsibility for prevention is usually separate from the emergency planning function. Legislation may often be required: for example, building regulations may need to be strengthened in earthquake zones; firearm legislation may reduce the likelihood of mass shootings.

Different types of disaster have differentiated impacts on health services. Some disasters result from a single event such as an earthquake or a fire, while others result from an ongoing problem, such as a pandemic or civil war. However, even a single event is likely to have enduring consequences, with a long 'recovery' phase in terms of the physical and psychological care of affected individuals, as well as in terms of social and economic disruption caused by the disaster. If the event has substantially disrupted health services, either by damage to buildings or by attrition of health service staff, rebuilding health services and the healthcare workforce will take time. This will be particularly true for the more fragile health systems affected by disasters in resource-poor communities.

Different types of disaster also vary in the specific demands that these place on responding health systems. Some pandemics (influenza, coronavirus) might require the capacity to ventilate affected patients, while in some large outbreaks or epidemics (Ebola, Lassa) this may be less important. Fire disasters, as mentioned, require the capacity to manage significant numbers of patients with burns. Earthquakes result in many crush injuries, with subsequent renal failure as a complication. Radiation sickness requires expert haematology care. Floods may create little demand for hospital care because survivors rarely have long-term physical problems. This simplified list makes clear that any major disaster will create a very wide range of problems to address.

In the UK, NHS England provides guidance to the health service on 'emergency preparedness, resilience and response' (EPRR) (NHS England, 2019), including a framework for EPRR, clinical guidance for major incidents, and an annual assurance process. The national agency for communicable disease emergencies is Public Health England, which provides extensive advice and support for local public health services, as well as laboratory services. A considerable part of the UK response to COVID-19 has been to emphasize the importance of changing individual behaviours, including hand washing and social distancing, using insights from behavioural science research. Often, the requirement to communicate risk in an emergency is for reassurance (Bradley et al., 2015). There is a considerable evidence base to design effective public communications in an emergency: this includes the message, who should convey it, the channel of communications to use, and so on.

Research should be a key part of disaster planning (Lurie et al., 2013). Rapidly conducted research can provide information concerning the scale and impact of an evolving emergency as well as developing, testing, and implementing evidence-based strategies for mitigation and control. Developing and scaling-up diagnostic tests, developing vaccines and other therapies, and evaluating their efficacy in well-designed trials, represent important research tasks that may require private sector participation.

16.3 Emergency preparation

The 'preparation' phase of the emergency response may overlap with the planning phase. It represents a process of rapid adaptation in the health system to cope with the expected surge in demand for services. Therrien et al. (2017) propose four aspects (the four 'S's) of surge capacity: 'staff'; 'stuff' (supplies and equipment); 'structures', including hospitals; and 'systems', including processes for decision making and collecting and disseminating information.

A key principle for staffing in a disaster response is to allocate staff to their normal roles, albeit perhaps in unusual circumstances. A disaster is not the time to call upon people to undertake unfamiliar, complex, or specialized tasks for the first time. Planning and preparation should ensure that staff receive training in key emergency tasks, which might include resuscitation following injuries, or ventilator training for the coronavirus pandemic. In the UK, a system of training has been developed for 'immediate care practitioners' (including doctors, nurses, and paramedics) who may provide voluntary major incident support to the existing emergency services. One difficulty in staffing for an ongoing disaster response is knowing how long staff can be expected to work. A shift of 14 hours or more may be reasonable on day one, but this is not sustainable as the scenario extends to weeks or months.

A large outbreak or pandemic may require mobilization of the public health workforce and reassignment to new tasks. Planning and preparation should maintain and update a contact list for all relevant staff. Group email systems have made this much easier in recent years; cascade calling has been used in the past and may still be an option. For example, the initiator calls ten people, each of whom then calls ten people; thus, two waves of calls can quickly reach a hundred people. In principle, this system can contact large numbers very quickly.

Preparing the supplies required to ensure that surge capacity matches expected demand is generally a task for healthcare providers. In the 2020 coronavirus epidemic, infectious disease modelling and analysis of real-time data helped to inform health services of expected levels and timing of peak demand for hospital and intensive care beds and requirements for ventilators and supplies of oxygen. Public health supplies may include vaccines and personal protective equipment, such as face masks. Continuity of the supply of medicines to a community may require attention in an extended or ongoing emergency. Preparations also need to focus on supply chains, distribution systems, and logistics to ensure that supplies are delivered to the places where they are needed, at the right time.

The 'structures' of a healthcare system include its buildings and other physical constructions. Each health provider must plan for optimal use of its own facilities, but the plan should also include co-opting extra facilities. Spaces such as large gyms and indoor recreation spaces may be required to provide shelter or to give extra capacity for patients; specialist and private sector hospitals may be asked, within the doctrine of 'do your normal job', to accept different types of patient.

Coordination of civil emergency responses between the public health system, health services, and local government is important. The decision to co-opt military personnel and resources is, for obvious reasons, taken at government level. The UK has a system of military aid to the civil authorities, known as MACA. Troops may be deployed to reinforce flood defences or deliver food parcels to remote communities, but sometimes more direct assistance to the health service is offered. This might include contributing to the logistics of distributing supplies or the rapid expansion of hospital capacity. In Italy, during the COVID-19 pandemic, troops were employed to transport deceased patients from overburdened mortuaries (Marsi, 2020). It is unusual for military personnel to be used in direct patient care roles, unless that is already normal practice.

'Systems' for command, communication, and coordination are crucial to the emergency response. 'Command' is best thought of as the system for making decisions. In the UK, the health system is dominated by a single public sector service. Elsewhere, multiple, sometimes competing, independent providers may need to collaborate and coordinate for the first time (Bradshaw, 2020). For acute emergencies in the UK, command structures are often labelled 'Gold' (strategic), 'Silver' (intermediate/district or regional), and 'Bronze' (local or tactical). The emergency plan needs to lay out, in advance, how agencies will collaborate in their decision making, who has authority to commit resources, and how decisions will be communicated quickly and effectively to those who need to know. In order to avoid potential rivalries over jurisdiction, the police force is usually regarded as the lead agency for most disasters.

One task for Gold control is to assemble expert advice, and to do so in advance. The UK government has a standing advisory group to provide scientific advice on emergencies. This high-level group employed a series of expert advisory groups to guide its decisions on the response to COVID-19 (UK Government, 2020), including mathematical modelling of the epidemic and evidence-based assessment of likely behaviour patterns among the general public. Ultimately, the selection of strategies for intervention and control become a matter for political decision. Sometimes, cultural awareness, from local knowledge or research, may be crucial for disease control. In the Ebola outbreak in West Africa in 2014, key questions related to the role of bats in transmission and, specifically, what kinds of wild meat were commonly consumed in the local population (Kümpel et al., 2015). Traditional funeral practices also contributed to the spread of disease and required reappraisal.

One important form of emergency preparation is to test or 'exercise' the plan. Such exercises vary in complexity from 'desk-top' exercises to test communication and command structures through to large-scale tests of hospital systems, with people simulating casualties. Most large hospitals will hold such exercises once every two or three years; a maximum interval of five years between exercises, though arbitrary, seems reasonable. Public health systems may also be tested, and the World Health Organization (2020) has produced training packages to help with the testing of local plans for aspects of pandemic influenza.

The value of such exercises depends on the level of their realism, which will benefit from expert input to the design (for example, with respect to the number, range, and types of injuries expected in a mass casualty incident), as well as from full engagement with the scenario by the responders. The 'post-exercise report' should be studied carefully and any lessons learned incorporated into a revised plan. Problems of communication between agencies are a recurring issue: for example, radios may not operate between, say, fire and ambulance services; and, more recently, interoperable computer networks have become problematical. Even simple emailing between one organization and another may be impossible due to data protection policies or a lack of logon and access rights.

The other benefit of exercises is to allow people who will work together in an emergency to become personally acquainted. Chess and Clarke (2007) provided an interesting analysis of organizational cooperation in the United States during the anthrax attacks of 2001.

16.4 Emergency response

The Prussian general Helmuth von Moltke declared that no plan survives contact with the enemy, or here, with the reality of an unfolding disaster. All plans, when enacted in real life, require active management and adaptation in response to changing situations and circumstances. Public health work is usually long-term and strategic rather than operational. Public health personnel may sometimes take a less prominent role in the response phase of a disaster, although this will not be the case for major infectious disease outbreaks and pandemics, or for chemical, environmental, and radiological hazards (Bradley et al., 2015). For a pandemic, such as COVID-19, a few highly specialist experts will advise government policy directly; the task for most of the public health workforce is to engage in developing and implementing national and local guidance, including testing, case finding, contact tracing, and mitigation measures.

One key decision is when to declare that an emergency exists and to initiate the plan. Mass casualty incidents declare themselves, but the decision may not be so clear-cut for communicable disease outbreaks. Surveillance systems help to give early warning and many countries now monitor influenza virus activity (UK Government, 2019). An epidemic is declared when a threshold is exceeded. For example, in the UK, the threshold is a rate of 200 people per 100,000 consulting a GP for 'influenza-like illness' in a week (UK Government, 2019). A more sophisticated approach is to monitor the rate of increase or uptick, which heralds the start of a major epidemic.

With epidemics from novel viruses such as SARS and COVID-19, our initial ignorance of parameters characterizing the risk of contagion and severity of illness may make judgements more difficult. The cases which come to notice first are likely to be more severe cases, causing us to overestimate the overall case fatality rate. In the absence of appropriate diagnostic tests, people with mild disease go unnoticed, leading to initial underestimation of the extent of the epidemic and rate of spread. We also need to know whether infection confers immunity. All of this makes it difficult to assess the likely course of the epidemic from preliminary data.

16.5 Recovery

Recovery is often overlooked in emergency plans. However, it takes time to get back to 'normal' after a disaster, and this phase needs active management. As a minimum, there will be a backlog of patients whose non-urgent treatment was deferred because of the greater urgency of the disaster victims. In addition, those who have suffered from the disaster will likely need a prolonged period of rehabilitation or ongoing treatment. At worst, as already noted, health service facilities may have been destroyed and need to be rebuilt; health service staff may have succumbed or migrated, and successors must be trained. Patients may need to be reassigned to other hospitals, which fared better; staff may need to be redeployed to cover critical vacancies.

16.6 Report

After the event, reports must be written to analyse the strengths and limitations of the emergency response. This may enable us to do better next time round, or perhaps to prepare for something we have never faced before. The COVID-19 pandemic prompted governments around the world to place unprecedented bans on gatherings, such as within schools and at sporting events—or almost unprecedented, since there was some experience to draw upon from the pandemic influenza of 1918/19 (Markel et al., 2007).

Immediate post-disaster reports can teach valuable lessons about the response phase—for example, problems of communication within and between teams at the King's Cross fire in 1987. Reports can also highlight the likely behaviours of the public in response to, for example, shelter-in-place versus evacuation orders (Mitchell et al., 2005). Even if no immediate report was possible, post-disaster epidemiology may improve our knowledge of the effects of radiation and chemicals in humans (Ozasa et al., 2017; Cullinan et al., 1997). Kulling et al. (2011) has provided a useful framework for the content of immediate post-disaster reports, including healthcare aspects.

16.7 Mental health and emergencies

Mental health concerns are an important dimension of the public health response to any emergency (World Health Organization, 2019). During a disaster or emergency, acute psychological distress is usually widespread. This can lead on to problems of anxiety, depression, post-traumatic stress syndrome, or substance abuse. Patients with pre-existing serious mental illnesses are especially vulnerable in disasters and emergencies. Planning for emergencies should address mental health and well-being, and ensure that the rights of the most vulnerable are protected. This may include promoting community self-help and social support through volunteer efforts; training key workers in psychological first aid, to provide immediate support to people experiencing acute distress; and ensuring access to primary healthcare for common mental disorders and to specialist interventions for those with more serious disorders (World Health Organization, 2019).

16.8 Service abroad

Responding to an emergency in a different country in need of assistance requires special mention. The key principle is that the incoming team should place absolutely no burden on the host country. Complete self-sufficiency of supplies, food, water, electricity, transport, and so on is almost impossible to achieve except perhaps through military deployments. Staff need protection against local communicable diseases, including appropriate vaccinations, and also pre-deployment briefing on hazards in the local environment including dangerous animals, heat, and/or cold stress. Bolton and Burkle (2013) have provided a useful summary. The local political situation is also important since incoming staff may have different social, economic, and cultural expectations than the local population, and intervention may raise the spectre of colonialism. Some thought needs to be given to the effect of providing different standards of care to disaster victims than can be provided in usual care settings in that environment. The situation is further complicated if the deployment is to an active conflict zone, but that is beyond the scope of this chapter. A number of organizations have risen to the challenges involved: Médecins Sans Frontières is among the best known.

16.9 Everyday resilience

Although the classic concept of a disaster or emergency is of a one-off event which threatens to overwhelm local facilities, Barasa et al. (2017) and Gilson et al. (2017) have proposed the concept of 'everyday resilience'. These authors make the point that, although we usually think of a disaster as a one-off shock to the system, and resilience as the capacity to rebound to normal afterwards, the reality for many global health systems is that they are constantly on the verge of being overwhelmed: dealing with this situation is an everyday task. Conversely, the everyday business of coping with disruptions and problems builds resilience—solutions are found and, more importantly, relationships are built. It is these relationships that keep systems performing when external or internal stresses increase. The concept of everyday resilience can be extended to networks of healthcare providers (Jessop, 2019).

Acknowledgements

I am very grateful to Allison Streetly and Martin Gulliford for valuable advice and contributions to this chapter.

References

Barasa, E.W., Cloete, K., & Gilson, L. (2017). From bouncing back, to nurturing emergence: reframing the concept of resilience in health systems strengthening. *Health Pol Plann*, 32, 91–94. doi: 10.1093/heapol/czx118

Bolton, P. & Burkle Jr, F.M. (2013). Emergency response. In: C. Guest, W. Ricciardi, I. Kawachi, & I. Lang (eds) *Oxford Handbook of Public Health Practice* (3rd edn). Oxford: Oxford University Press.

Bradley, N., Meara, J., & Murray, V. (2015). Principles of public health emergency response for acute environmental, chemical, and radiation incidents. In R. Detels, M. Gulliford, Q.A. Karim, & C.C. Tan (eds) *Oxford Textbook of Global Public Health* (6th edn). Oxford: Oxford University Press.

Bradshaw, P. (2020). Midnight family review—an alarming look at Mexico's ambulance cowboys. *Guardian*, 19 February 2020. Available at: https://www.theguardian.com/film/2020/feb/19/midnight-family-review-luke-lorentzen-mexico-ambulance-documentary [accessed 26 March 2020].

Chess, C. & Clarke, L. (2007). Facilitation of risk communication during the anthrax attacks of 2001: the organizational backstory. *Am J Public Health*, 97, 1578–1583. doi.org/10.2105/AJPH.2006.099267

Cullinan, T., Acquilla, S., & Dhara, V.R. (1997). Respiratory morbidity 10 years after the Union Carbide gas leak at Bhopal: a cross sectional survey. *BMJ*, 314, 338.

Gilson, L., et al. (2017) Everyday resilience in district health systems: emerging insights from the front lines in Kenya and South Africa. *BMJ Glob Health*, 2, e000224. doi: 10.1136/bmjgh-2016-000224

Jessop, E. (2019). Resilience in rare disease networks. *Ann Ist Super Sanità*, 55(3), 292–295.

Kulling, P., Birnbaum, M., Murray, V., & Rockenschaub, G. (2011). (A58) Guidelines for reports on health crises and critical health events—a tool for the development of disaster medicine research. *Prehosp Disaster Med*, 26(Suppl 1), S16. doi: 10.1017/S1049023X11000653

Kümpel, N.F., Cunningham, A.A., Fa, J.E., Jones, J.P.G., Rowcliffe, J.M., & Milner–Gulland, E.J. (2015). Ebola and bushmeat: myth and reality. *NWFP Update 5: Bushmeat*. Rome: Food and Agriculture Organization of the United Nations. Available at: http://forestry.fao.msgfocus.com/q/15RgxaesHEFDyqbhiv/wv [accessed 4 May 2020].

Lurie, N., Manolio, T., Patterson, A.P., Collins, F., & Frieden, T. (2013). Research as a part of public health emergency response. *New Engl J Med*, 368(13), 1251–1255.

Markel, H., et al. (2007). Nonpharmaceutical interventions implemented by US cities during the 1918–1919 influenza pandemic. *JAMA*, 298(6), 644–654.

Marsi, F. (2020). Army drafted in to help move corpses from 'Italy's Wuhan'. *Independent*, 19 March 2020. Available at: https://www.independent.co.uk/news/world/europe/coronavirus-italy-army-deaths-corpses-bodies-bergamo-cases-a9411401.html [accessed 26 March 2020].

Mitchell, J., et al. (2005). *Evacuation behavior in response to the Graniteville, South Carolina, chlorine spill*. Available at: https://hazards.colorado.edu/uploads/basicpage/qr178.pdf [accessed 27 March 2020].

NHS England. (2019). *Emergency preparedness, resilience and response (EPRR)*. Available at: https://www.england.nhs.uk/ourwork/eprr/ [accessed 28 March 2020].

Ozasa, K., Grant, E.J., & Kodama, K. (2018). Japanese legacy cohorts: The Life Span Study atomic bomb survivor cohort and survivors' offspring. *J Epidemiol*, 28(4), 162–169. doi.org/10.2188/jea.JE20170321

Roberts, L. & Brennan, R. (2015). Emergency public health and humanitarian assistance in the twenty-first century. In: R. Detels, M. Gulliford, Q.A. Karim, & C.C. Tan (eds) *Oxford Textbook of Global Public Health* (6th edn). Oxford: Oxford University Press.

Therrien, M.C., Normandin, J.M., & Denis, J.L. (2017). Bridging complexity theory and resilience to develop surge capacity in health systems. *J Health Organiz Manag*, 31, 96–109. doi.org/10.1108/JHOM-04-2016-0067

UK Government. (2019). *Sources of UK flu data: influenza surveillance in the UK*. Available at: https://www.gov.uk/guidance/sources-of-uk-flu-data-influenza-surveillance-in-the-uk [accessed 26 March 2020].

UK Government. (2020). *Scientific Advisory Group for Emergencies (SAGE): coronavirus (COVID-19) response*. Available at: https://www.gov.uk/government/groups/scientific-advisory-group-for-emergencies-sage-coronavirus-covid-19-response [accessed 26 March 2020].

United Nations Office for Disaster Risk Reduction (UNDRR). (2020). *United Nations Office for Disaster Risk Reduction: terminology*. Geneva, Switzerland: UNDRR. Available at: https://www.undrr.org/terminology [accessed 28 March 2020].

World Health Organization. (2019). *Mental health in emergencies*. Geneva, Switzerland: World Health Organization. Available at: https://www.who.int/news-room/fact-sheets/detail/mental-health-in-emergencies [accessed 29 March 2020].

World Health Organization. (2020). *Training: welcome to the WHO emergency risk communication learning course* Available at: https://www.who.int/risk-communication/training/en/ [accessed 26 March 2020].

17
Concluding remarks

Edmund Jessop and Martin Gulliford

17.1 Introduction

In this book we have focused on the here and now, but what might the future hold for healthcare public health? Prediction is always unwise, but perhaps we can venture some general observations. Certainly, demographic and economic constraints will play their part—it seems inevitable that both the amount and the shape of healthcare systems will be stretched by increasing numbers of old people, even as the definition of 'old age' is itself stretched. Increasing specialization in medical and other disciplines will progressively fragment care. Recent advances in genomics will change our concepts of disease.

17.2 Demographic change

Let us consider demographics and economics first. In most public healthcare systems, taxes on the young pay for care of the old. In a healthcare economy, it matters not just how many old people there are, but also how many young people there are in the workforce. Some jurisdictions, such as Hong Kong and Bulgaria, have increasingly inverted population pyramids—the old outnumber the young—due to declining birth rates (Hong Kong) or outward migration (Bulgaria). In such places, the tax base for funding public healthcare is shrinking as the demand for healthcare increases.

Policy responses to this problem have included personal healthcare budgets, provident systems, restrictions on eligibility, and restrictions on public-sector provision. Restrictions on eligibility provision are contentious, particularly in jurisdictions such as the UK, with a long history of almost unlimited services. There is general agreement that cosmetic surgery should not be funded by the tax payer—or, more precisely, 'aesthetic' surgery should not, since cosmetic surgery may be required for the gross disfigurements of congenital disorder, trauma, or cancer resections. Restrictions on fertility treatment are more controversial, as are treatments for sexual dysfunctions, whilst almost everyone (other than those responsible for staying within budget) objects to restrictions on cataract surgery or hip replacement.

Restrictions lead to debate about the appropriate target for healthcare services. What is their scope? Some jurisdictions use the concept of 'all medically necessary services'; others prefer 'appropriate' care. The NHS Management Executive (1991)

Edmund Jessop and Martin Gulliford, *Concluding remarks* In: *Healthcare Public Health*. Edited by: Martin Gulliford and Edmund Jessop, Oxford University Press (2020). © Oxford University Press. DOI: 10.1093/oso/9780198837206.003.0017.

defined 'need' as the 'ability to benefit from health care'. However, these definitions are somewhat circular—anything treatable should be treated. In this debate, the famous definition of health as a state of complete physical, mental, and social well-being becomes deeply unhelpful. If anything which increases physical, mental, or social well-being is the legitimate target of a healthcare system, then all human activity, including a nice holiday somewhere sunny, is to be included.

The American State of Oregon developed an interesting public process to define which procedures should be covered by the State's Medicaid programme (Perry,2011)[1]—but it has not been widely copied. Most jurisdictions muddle through with a mixture of public- and private-coverage decisions, some based on explicit values and some on emotional response. All of this is frustrating for the evidence-based and scientific planner, but it is probably inevitable in any political economy.

In 1980, Fries introduced the notion (or perhaps the hope?) of compression of morbidity, stating that it 'occurs if the age at first appearance of aging manifestations and chronic disease symptoms can increase more rapidly than life expectancy' (Fries, 2005). If completely true, increasing numbers of old people would not increase the requirement for healthcare: people live longer but have a shorter period of age-related frailty and dependency. In many countries, it is already clear that people are increasingly healthy in old age: a typical 75 year old is more active and more healthy today than in 1980, and a number of studies have documented decreasing age-specific prevalence of major diseases such as cardiovascular disease and dementia. Hence the view arises that 'old age' may itself need a new definition, acknowledged by the UK government as the age of entitlement to a state 'old age' pension is steadily increased. However, the compression of morbidity has been relative, not absolute, and so the total amount of healthcare needed by old people is greater now than in 1980.

One interesting question is the extent to which the multiple impairments of old age should require us to change the categories we use to classify disease. On the one hand, people of any age require prompt diagnosis followed by specific treatment for specific diseases: interventions directed at minimizing the impact of an occluded artery or a broken bone are as relevant to a 90 year old as to patients 40 or 50 years younger. On the other hand, frailty may dictate a different approach to managing the whole person: optimizing functional ability may be more important than controlling multiple disease processes. Capturing this change in perspective has implications for the way we secure information about patients. The International Classification of Diseases (ICD) has served us well for over a century. It is the dominant classification for routine mortality statistics and for episodes of hospital care worldwide; it is however notoriously poor at capturing information about disease severity, disabilities, and impairments. Classifications of impairment and disability are available but they are not used in routine data systems. An alternative approach is to use existing datasets

---

[1] Oregon put a list of hundreds of procedures into priority order, and drew a line: above the line, the service or procedure would be reimbursed, below the line, it would not. In 1995, for example, the top 581 out of 745 procedures were covered.

to construct ad hoc indices of comorbidity or frailty (the Charlson Index is probably the most famous of these), but such indices are limited in scope and accuracy. A more radical rethink would be required to enable us to track routinely the functional status of patients receiving healthcare.

17.3 Complex pathways

The healthcare process is increasingly complex. The classic model envisages a simple linear pathway for patients from primary care to the local general hospital, and thence to regional specialist care. However, the pathway now offers many other options and routes. At the level of primary care, patients can consult a traditional general practitioner (GP) or family doctor, but they can also turn to telephone advice services such as NHS Direct, walk-in centres, and self-care (with or without instructions from the internet). A GP may refer patients to a variety of healthcare services other than the local hospital, such as physiotherapy, weight-loss services, smoking cessation support, counselling, and so on. The local hospital may deploy remote monitoring or telemedicine services; and the whole notion of a 'general' hospital seems increasingly dated. Referral management systems, aimed at controlling demand and activity, disrupt the traditional relationship between a referring GP and a hospital consultant. In the fields of mental health and palliative care, outreach services from the hospital may serve patients at home or at local clinics. Within the specialist centre, increasing subspecialization is producing, for example, skull-base surgeons and epilepsy surgeons within neurosurgery, and cardiologists who specialize in rhythm, muscle, or valve disorders. Particularly in small jurisdictions, patients may need to travel to other countries for treatment.

All of this complexity carries implications for both planners and patients. For patients, increasing complexity reinforces disadvantage—navigating a complex system requires cognitive, physical, and financial resources. Well-educated, affluent patients can learn how to move through the system to get the care they need; they can also travel to receive it. Less able patients may not be aware of what is available, or not know how to access it. In principle, the National Health Service in Britain is rooted in the general practitioner having a one-to-one relationship with his or her patients: all you have to do is visit your GP and the GP will take it from there. This is still the ideal, and still the reality in a few places, but it seems increasingly difficult to sustain.

For healthcare public health, the challenge is to understand this complexity, or at least to notice it. Mapping patient journeys through the system, noticing the delays and duplications and blocks, requires considerably sophisticated data systems at a time when tracking identifiable patients is increasingly hampered by data protection legislation. At its simplest, the healthcare public health task is to be aware of just how complex the system has become—and to remind others of that fact. It is all too easy to focus on one's own part of any system. The danger is that an apparently helpful change or modification, made in ignorance of the wider picture, becomes deeply dysfunctional to the system as a whole.

Responses to complexity have included innovations such as the 'one-stop shop', to meet all of the patient's needs in a single visit, or a 'single number phone call'. Care managers or care coordinators, and, more recently, patient advocates, may help. However, the research evidence on their effect is not encouraging. We probably need to accept that complexity is, to a greater or lesser extent, a feature of life in the twenty-first century; it is the price we pay for the astonishing increase in treatment options for a huge range of diseases over the past two or three decades.

17.4 Nosology

The work of defining, classifying, and categorizing disease—nosology—can fairly be claimed as a task for epidemiology, and thus public health. We touched earlier on some aspects of old age and multiple morbidity which challenge our thinking about the classification of ill health. Another challenge to our concepts of disease comes from developments in genomics and cell biology. The complex relationship between genotype and phenotype means that the same 'disease'—that is, the same pattern of symptoms and functional impairments—may arise from many different mutations in a single gene, or from mutations in apparently unrelated genes. In some situations, the specific mutation may be strongly predictive of early-onset severe disease or of late-onset mild disease. This opens the way to screening programmes, prophylactic treatments, and a variety of healthcare interventions.

However, a person with no detectable signs or symptoms may be found to have a mutation which, in other people, is clearly associated with disease. Indeed, identical (monozygotic) twins have been described who have the same mutation in the same gene but hugely different phenotypes. This is much more problematical for screening and prophylaxis. What should we do if we cannot predict whether an individual, known to have a particular mutation, is likely to develop severe, disabling disease or something almost undetectable clinically? It also raises the wider question of what counts as a disease. Should we label people with a known disease-causing mutation as having the disease, even if they remain asymptomatic?

We may wonder if any of this matters. In the world of hypercholesterolaemia, there is a doctrine of 'treat the phenotype, counsel the genotype': if the patient has a high cholesterol, use standard treatment algorithms, regardless of the genetic mutation which has led to that hypercholesterolaemia. Identifying a precise mutation is irrelevant. However, mutation-specific drugs are now being developed for some diseases, and then it certainly does matter what the underlying mutation is. This is already relevant in treating people with, for example, Duchenne muscular dystrophy or Fabry disease. Likewise in the world of cancer therapeutics, a number of highly active monoclonal antibody treatments target molecules which are expressed on the cell surface. The question then is not whether the patient has lung cancer or skin cancer, but whether the cancer cell is expressing the antigen PD-L1. Certainly, these developments are outpacing the ability of public health data systems to keep track: if the clinical and treatment classification is based on molecular biology not anatomy, ICD cannot cope.

17.5 The future of healthcare public health

What does all this mean for the public health workforce? Perhaps the best way to address this question is by considering the effect of these changes on the knowledge, skills, and attitudes required to practice healthcare public health.

In the area of knowledge, it seems that a basic understanding of information systems and of genomics will be important. The complexity of healthcare pathways discussed earlier, and problems of classification and coding, will lead to new developments. Information and statistics from routine systems can never be taken at face value—errors and artefacts can arise at all stages of data capture, coding, and classification; expertise is required to locate the truth. For high-stakes decisions, this probably means seeking the advice of experts in public health intelligence, but such experts are in short supply, overworked, and difficult to access. Hence all workers in healthcare public health will need a good working knowledge of the main features of the major information systems. Special expertise is of course also required to design and implement new information systems.

The same applies to public health genomics. This is a highly technical area and expertise is required to interpret both research studies and routine reports from, for example, whole-genome sequencing. Again, we might envisage a basic grounding for all public health workers, with a few topic experts to advise on high-stakes decisions and to advance the science.

In the area of skills, it is right to highlight the importance of strong interpersonal skills. Reducing the increasing complexity of healthcare pathways and simplifying the flow, for the benefit of patients, will require a large number of diverse agencies and personalities to work together. Public health has no monopoly on wisdom or skill in this area, but on the other hand, interagency work is so much a part of all aspects of public health work that we certainly have something to offer and should not be falsely modest about that.

The area of attitudes may perhaps be less affected by the changes we have discussed. The enduring requirement in all public health work is a concern for the underserved—for population coverage and for inequality. Change and increasing complexity always favour the well-resourced: the rich and powerful, those with cognitive resources from a good education, those with financial resources to step outside the public sector, those with the selfconfidence to demand a response from public services. The public health worker must constantly seek to redress that imbalance between the well-off and the less well-off, to ensure that the latter gain fully from all the benefits of scientific advance and service change.

References

Fries, J. (2005). The compression of morbidity. *Milbank Q*, 83(4), 801–823.

NHS Management Executive. (1991). *Assessing Health Care Needs*. London: Department of Health.

Perry, P.A. & Hotze, T. (2011). Oregon's experiment with prioritizing public health care services. *Virtual Mentor*, 13(3), 241–247.

Index

Note: tables, figures, and boxes are indicated by an italic *t*, *f*, and *b* following the page number.

For the benefit of digital users, indexed terms that span two pages (e.g., 52–53) may, on occasion, appear on only one of those pages.